PRAISE FOR
DEATH OF THE DIET

"Delightful read using a proven approach to motivating behavior change. Machowsky understands that achieving long-term results is a process determined by the many decisions we face day-to-day. *Death of the Diet* is all about identifying the fork in the decision-tree and enabling you to choose the right branch using two key qualities for success: happiness and purpose. I highly recommend this book to health professionals and consumers alike."

Marissa Beck, MS, RD, Director of Wellness at NextJump, Inc.

"A fresh perspective on making great nutrition a reality. This book is full of easy steps you can incorporate immediately to make a big impact on how you will look and feel for years to come."

Amanda Carlson-Phillips, MS, RD, CSSD,
VP of Nutrition & Research at Athletes' Performance

"*Death of the Diet* is a quick read; full of inspirational advice for those who want to not only make changes to their daily eating habits and physical activities, but also adopt a healthy lifestyle for the long haul. Highly recommend for solid, real-life advice."

Dr. Nancy Collins, PhD, RD, LD/N, Founder of Nutrition411.com

"Jason provides simple, realistic solutions for maintaining optimum health based on his experience, research and client feedback. Time and time again *Death of the Diet* offers examples of how exercise and nutrition work together to achieve and sustain desired results. Simply put, the book provides a comprehensive, logical approach to tackling a lifelong demon for so many people."

Pete Draovitch, MS, PT, ATC, CSCS,
Hospital for Special Surgery & Author of Complete Conditioning for Golf

"This is by far the most comprehensive book on losing weight I've read. If losing weight is about "just eating healthfully and exercising" why don't we all do it? Because it's hugely psychological. *Death of the Diet* helps tremendously because not only does it teach you what to do, but also how to implement it consistently – the missing key to long-term results."

Adam Gilbert, Founder of MyBodyTutor.com

"Jason walks the walk and talks the talk. It is wonderful to get pearls of wisdom from someone who has 'been there, done that' in weight management and decided to make their career out of it by becoming a Registered Dietitian. *Death of the Diet* provides sound strategies for successful weight management – once and for all!"

Dr. Felicia Stoler, RD, DCN, FACSM, Author of Living Skinny in Fat Genes

DEATH OF THE DIET

EIGHT EASY HABITS TO GET THE BODY YOU WANT, PERMANENTLY

JASON MACHOWSKY, MS, RD, CSCS

wellness

NOTICE & DISCLAIMER

This book is intended as a reference volume only, not as a medical manual. The information provided in this book is designed to help you make informed decisions about your health and wellness. It is not intended to be a substitute for any medical treatments prescribed by your doctor. If you suspect you have a medical problem, seek medical help promptly.

You should get your doctor's approval before starting any new exercise or dietary programs. The exercise and dietary suggestions in this book are not intended as a substitute for any exercise routine or dietary regimen that may have been prescribed by your doctor.

The information in this book is not meant to replace proper exercise training. All forms of exercise pose some inherent risks and the writer advises readers to take full responsibility for their safety. Be sure not to take risks beyond your level of experience, training and fitness. The writer, editors and publisher are not responsible for negative consequences, injuries or harm that may result from improper use of this book.

Mention of specific companies, organizations or authorities in this book does not imply endorsement by the author or publisher and vice versa. Internet addresses and telephone numbers provided in this book were accurate at the time it went to press.

Every effort made to denote third-party trademarks, trade names or service names with initial capitalization in the text or through direct references.

www.JasonMachowsky.com
www.DeathoftheDiet.com

Copies of this book can be purchased in bulk quantities at reduced rates.
Contact: info@jasonmachowsky.com

Book and cover design by: Duolit, LLC
Editing by: Rebecca Meyer
Indexing by: Dan Connolly
Author Photo by: Michelle Timek
Training Photos taken by Rebecca Meyer at Hamilton Health and Fitness, Jersey City, NJ
ISBN: 978-0-9886873-0-1
e-ISBN: 978-0-9886873-1-8
Library of Congress Control Number: 2012922443

To my parents, who said I could do anything if I put my mind to it.

To Becca, my love and my editor – in print and in life.

ACKNOWLEDGEMENTS

Without my family, friends, colleagues and clients, this book wouldn't exist. I decided to make this list chronological, because it was the easiest way for my former engineer brain to craft it:

Many thanks to my parents for raising this Jersey boy well. Lauren, thanks for kindly forcing me to look inside myself for what I really wanted out of life in 2005. Thanks to my Deloitte colleagues for being so supportive during my personal transformation. Tyler, I appreciate you sticking with me and inspiring me to take life by the horns.

My time at Teachers College and Equinox were transformational. Lora, thank you for being a constant source of guidance and positivity. To Marissa, Jesse and all of my TC classmates, I've learned from all of you. To Dwayne, Jon, Jemimah, Jeremy and all of my other Equinox colleagues from 92nd St. and Columbus Circle, you've successfully challenged me to put my book smarts into action.

California dreamin' – thank you Lori, Brooke and the entire PDC dietetic internship crew for providing me with my first true dietitian experiences and helping me feel at home when I was so far away.

To my colleagues at Hospital for Special Surgery – Polly, Jamie, Kara, Mike and the entire rehab team – and my Jersey City peeps – HHF & Crew, Sarah & FlorYoga – my experiences with you have helped hone this book into what it is. Thanks to everyone who gave me a chance to practice my nascent writing skills – Michelle & the Food Network Healthy Eats blog, Nancy & Nutrition411.com.

To my clients – you are the reason why this book has come to be, and anyone who benefits from it has you to thank.

To everyone who has helped make this book readable, I can't thank you enough. To the kind staff at the Grove St. Starbucks in Jersey City: thanks for not throwing me out. To Liz, Jon, Breanna, Adam and Dwayne: thanks for reading and providing feedback on my unwieldy first draft – your patience and perseverance is appreciated. To my expert design team: Chip, Kim, Toni, Shannon and Dan, thanks for helping me execute my vision of a book that looks good inside and out. To the best editor a man could ever ask for, Becca, you molded my words into a comprehensible piece of writing.

And last, but certainly not least, to my friends and family who've supported me throughout my life. A kind word, a helping hand, a hug. I feel honored and blessed to call all of you my support system. I hope this book lives up to your faith in me.

TABLE OF
CONTENTS

FOREWORD

MY FAMILY'S JOURNEY TO HEALTH AND WELLNESS

B efore delving into the topics, experiences and thoughts in this book that reflect who I am today, I would like to give you a glimpse into the person who I was; this entire journey started from there. For the first eighteen years of my life, I was relatively inactive and did not pay much attention to how I ate (like most kids). I couldn't stick to any sport; I would start, grow frustrated at my inability to perform, and then stop participating. Taekwondo, basketball, baseball, soccer and more. You name it, I tried it…and quit. I felt that I couldn't play any sport well…so I just did nothing at all.

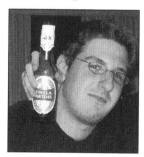

BEFORE: A FEW TOO MANY STELLAS EVERY WEEK.

As a result, I was always that "husky" kid, self-conscious about taking his shirt off at the pool and absolutely dreading the "Presidential Fitness Challenge" tests every year in gym class. To boot, I had to visit a chiropractor regularly throughout middle school and high school to treat chronic headaches that sometimes caused such severe pain that I didn't

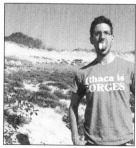

AFTER: A BIT SVELTER. I CREDIT THE APPLE.

1

want to move for hours. Of course, little did I know that many of these issues related to my fitness level (or lack thereof).

My first taste of fitness came in college when I lifted weights and did cardio on an on-and-off basis. While my headaches vanished with this increased activity, my extra weight did not. I gained and lost fifteen pounds multiple times during my college years due to my inconsistent eating and activity habits. Every time the scale tipped over 200 pounds (a result of sitting for hours studying, lots of late night snacks, etc.), it was my mental cue to eat less and exercise a lot more for a few weeks until I got back down to 185 pounds. I remember working out thirteen days in a row during one of these "health binges." But of course, intensity like that is not sustainable, so the cycle repeated itself.

After graduation, I started a corporate job that involved sitting most of the day, eating out regularly and going to client dinners often. While I got to eat and drink well during these years, my fitness, energy and personal life began to suffer. Constant travel made it challenging to maintain relationships with friends, family and my girlfriend, which led to even more stress and more eating. By the end of 2004, I was overweight, tipping the scale at about 205 pounds, unhappy in my corporate job and dealing with a difficult break-up. My days were full of deadlines and commitments that did not motivate me. I was not enjoying my life because of my work and my weight. I knew *something* had to change.

For the first time, I started considering what I wanted out of my life. I knew I wanted to help others, as I had always enjoyed teaching and volunteering. But I wasn't helping anyone through my job at the time…well, aside from helping Fortune 500 companies make more money. I wanted to start by helping myself become the person I always wanted to be…and feel. So I decided to start making decisions for myself and savoring life by becoming more active and eating better.

In 2005, I lost about 35 pounds by gradually learning and acting on all the information I could find about weight loss, proper nutrition and physical activity. Due to my engineering background, I am very numbers-oriented, so I decided to keep track of my calories and physical activity. Then, I adjusted my routines based on the results I was getting…or not getting. Looking back at my progression, I realize that my own health, fitness and weight loss success was the result of a series of changes to my habits over time:

1. **Before making any changes, I first kept a food journal to track my current eating habits.** When I reviewed the journal, I was amazed to see that I was actually under-eating for my daily calorie needs. My metabolism had stalled and my energy was low, especially at the end of the day. This made getting to the gym after work a seriously difficult task! I increased my meal frequency (Habit #1) by adding mid-morning and mid-afternoon snacks, which gave me more energy for the day, and for better workouts.

2. **Rather than flip-flopping between different numbers of workouts each week, I committed to going to the gym three days a week.** I only increased my workout frequency after steadily attending three times a week for a couple of months. (Habit #6)

3. **I made it a point to reduce how often or how much I indulged during the workday and on weekends with friends.** I began reserving my indulgences for the times when I really wanted them, which was still at least a couple of times per week at the occasional client dinner and birthday party. (Habit #5)

4. **I started making sure I stood up and moved more throughout the day.** I realized I could easily go hours without getting out of my chair, so I made it a point to get up and drink more water. It pulled double duty: I got up to drink more water. Then I had to get up again to pee it out. (Habit #4 and #7)

   Note: The Easy Eight Habits have corresponding numbers, described in detail in Chapter 7. All habit numbers referenced above are related to those specific habits.

My transformation was slow, choppy and filled with temptations. Did I miss workouts? You bet. Did I still occasionally eat too much at client dinners or have a few too many beers with friends? Yep. But every time I got tripped up,

I reflected on why I was making the change. I no longer wanted to be self-conscious when I took off my shirt and I wanted to finally look the way I acted… energetic and happy. My weight loss journey took ten months of imperfect, but consistent, steps towards health and happiness.

This was the first transformational experience that led me to my current profession as a Registered Dietitian, personal trainer and wellness coach. The second and most important transformational experience was helping one of the most important people in my life: my mom.

MY MOM'S JOURNEY TO WELLNESS

My mom was your typical, chronic yo-yo dieter, weighing between 130 and 200 pounds many times since her twenties. You name the diet and she probably tried it. I recall seeing her weight fluctuate quite a few times during my childhood, and also a very scary bout of pancreatitis that sent her to the hospital. The likely culprit in that sickness? After being vegetarian for a number of years, stress had caused my mom to start binge eating on a variety of processed, high fat foods like spare ribs and doughnuts.

After this episode, my mom went vegetarian (no meat, though she still eats fish, eggs and dairy) for good, but still continued to deal with weight issues. That is, until 2006 when I had the privilege of working with her to determine a plan that allowed my mom to finally take control of her weight for the first time ever in her adult life—at the age of 56! It was, and still is, one of the most inspiring feelings I've ever had. I asked her to provide a recollection of her own experiences of the transformation and her life since:

"All my adult life my weight would yo-yo, as much as twenty pounds in a single year. When the year wasn't a 'successful' yo-yo year, I would just gain weight; in the mid-1990s, I reached 203lbs. The idea of exercise, although not foreign to me, was never a constant part of my life. When I was 56 years old, Jason worked with me to create an eating plan based on my current habits: foods that I liked, reasonable portions and five times a day.

With my eating in order, he then worked with me to create several workout routines based on many of the exercises and machines I already knew. Jason showed me how to do the few new exercises I had never done before, but practicing involved doing it on my own and occasionally asking the trainers at my gym for help. I added the workouts one-by-one to my routine until it became an easy rotation. I was finally working out consistently and keep my metabolism working at peak efficiency!

Jason was always there to give me encouragement and advice during my weight loss; and he's also been there to help since. I reached my goal of staying between 135 and 145 pounds in 2006. And I'm still in that range six years later in 2012, the longest I've ever maintained a steady weight in my adult life.

Once on the road to health, you just look for more ways to get healthier. I now find that I miss going to the gym if some event in my life prevents me from getting to my workout. And I'm always looking for ways to improve my eating habits, but still listening to my body for feedback. You are never too old to start a healthy lifestyle, you just need the right person to give guidance and support, and for me, that was Jason because he never told me what to do, but helped me to discover that what I knew, inside myself, would work for me.

I wasn't always sure he knew what he was talking about...like when I hit a plateau, and he suggested that I increase my caloric intake for a couple of weeks, and then go back to my usual calories because my body had begun to believe I was starving, and had begun to hold on to weight...but he was right. I also knew that he had faith in me, and that I would do what was necessary to overcome the frustration of having my weight loss plateau, and that helped me to have faith in myself.

Over the years, there have been times of stress when I thought that I wanted to go back to food to make me feel better. What I found is that what I learned about my relationship with food during my weight loss has become a part of me. I deeply know that it will not help my situation to misuse food, and it is not a valid option for me anymore.

I also know, if I need encouragement, I can go to my health coach, Jason, for support. It's also true that the times that I have 'slipped' and eaten *more than I should, or if I have eaten what I know to be a poor nutritional choice, the food no longer really tastes as good as I imagined it, or it gives me an upset stomach. Knowing there is someone to encourage and support me is a wonderful thing, but the fact that most of the time I don't need outside help to stay on track is even better. I have gotten in touch with my body, and we actually communicate with each other."*

After feeling the success of my effort and my mom's, I knew that I'd found my true calling and the best use of my analytical engineering abilities: working with people to craft their own healthy lifestyles through their eating and physical activity habits. So, I left my corporate job to go back to school and learn how to effectively use movement and nutrition to enable others to live their best lives. I never looked back.

Since then I've been able to motivate and guide many others in their pursuit of maximizing their lives and happiness through their physical activity and eating habits. This book lays out the primary lesson I have learned: *small changes performed consistently over time will outperform crash diets and exercise fads in the long run, every time.*

DEFINING YOUR JOURNEY TO WELLNESS

After sharing two personal treks to wellness, I hope you feel inspired to start your own journey from where you are right now. The biggest commitment you can make at this point is to yourself. And written commitments often mean more than fleeting thoughts. So read the pledge on the next page and take a minute to consider each of the points. When you feel ready, sign it, photocopy it and post it somewhere that you'll see it every day.

MY PLEDGE TO PERMANENT CHANGE
FOR PERMANENT RESULTS:

1. *I will take full advantage of all that this book has to offer by reading it with an open mind.*

2. *I will make an honest effort to participate in all aspects of the chapters and activities to the best of my abilities.*

3. *I truly desire to improve my health, fitness and/or weight and am willing to put in the effort and persistence needed to achieve it, no matter how long it takes.*

4. *I believe that I have the power, ability and resiliency to achieve my goals regardless of the obstacles I may encounter.*

5. *I am willing to face and overcome the roadblocks and fears that may stand between me and a healthier, more fulfilling life.*

6. *I am willing to take an objective look at my current eating and physical activity habits, accept where I am at this moment in time and look to create improvements that will get me from where I am to where I want to be.*

7. *As I learn more, I will create a plan that I know I can reliably stick to and improve upon over time.*

8. *If I feel that I need help or guidance on a particular subject or activity, I will actively seek it out.*

9. *I will look to those that I trust, including myself, for support and positivity. I will not be a source of doubt or negativity.*

10. *I will share my vision of life, health and weight improvement with those that I know will support me and my mission.*

11. *I believe that there is no such thing as failure, only feedback.*

12. *I will strive to improve every day.*

_____
SIGNATURE

_____
DATE

CHAPTER 1

THE SECRETS TO PERMANENT HEALTH AND FITNESS

Are you satisfied with your current health, fitness or weight? Then you don't need to read this book. For everyone else, you are holding a book that shows you how to make small, sustainable adjustments to create permanent changes in your eating, physical activity and lifestyle habits; the result will be lasting improvements in your health, fitness and weight.

EVOLUTION OF *DEATH OF THE DIET* AND THE EASY EIGHT HABITS

When I first started working with clients in my newfound profession, I had this grand idea that I could work with people for a few months, give them an exercise and nutrition plan and *poof* they become svelte and fit. Think of it as "body engineering."

I was great at working with my clients to figure out what they wanted to accomplish (lose weight, get toned, etc.) and creating a plan to get them there. I even asked them what their food and training preferences were and tried to work with their schedules. However, my elaborate nutrition and fitness plans, designed to make a positive overhaul to their health, fitness or weight, often went unexecuted. Hours of my effort, collecting dust in a desk drawer or lost somewhere in an inbox.

Week in and week out I would see my clients, and their bodies never changed. I was doing all I could, training them two to three times a week. Did they get stronger? Yep. Did they gain balance? You bet. Better endurance? That too. But they rarely lost the weight or achieved the physique they wanted. It was a frustrating experience for all of us.

I thought that my client's success rested on me and I had to give them more and more education until they got the results. I kept racking my brain for what advice or resources I needed to provide to make the difference. But no matter how hard I pushed, most people didn't change. I slowly came to the conclusion that I could not take ultimate responsibility for my clients' weight or health because I could not control their decisions during the other 165 hours of the week (i.e. doing "homework" workouts and eating nutritious food).

After realizing this, my view of the entire health professional/client relationship changed. I had everything backwards; the crucial variable in body engineering was not any of my recommendations. It was my client. A plan is useless unless it is performed consistently.

But clients can't be controlled like a computer program. I can't force feed them carrots and avocado (though I've considered it). Humans are subject to inconveniences like long days at work, unforeseen meetings, cravings, temptations, emotional eating, social eating and more. Some health professionals call it non-compliance. I just call it dealing with life. I realized that rather than trying to make my client conform to a plan (even one initially based on their perceived preferences), I had to continuously tweak the plan to conform to my client's situation and needs.

And the revelations didn't stop there. What my client and I both also failed to realize is: what we *think* we want (our health, fitness or weight change goals) isn't always what we *truly* want. Many times we've never taken the time to sit, think and clarify what we want or *why* we want it. We just know that we don't want to be where we currently are. So we do anything and everything possible to get away from our current situation, without regard for our ultimate destination.

Upon reflection, we may not necessarily want to put in the effort required to get the results we think we want. Do you really want to be 6% body fat or weigh what you did before your first pregnancy if it means that you can only eat oatmeal, salads and grilled chicken most days, exercise five days per week and have only one dessert *per week*? To achieve long-term success, you must gradually reconcile the differences between the results you want and the permanent changes you're willing to make to get there.

These realizations led me to build a nutrition and training approach revolving around four main ideas:

1. CURRENT RESULTS = CURRENT EATING HABITS + CURRENT PHYSICAL ACTIVITY HABITS + CURRENT LIFESTYLE HABITS:

You must take an honest and non-judgmental look at your current habits and results to see what choices have led you to your current health, fitness or weight. Once you use basic assessments to understand where you are and what's caused you to get there, you can start deciding where to make improvements. For example, if you are currently gaining unwanted weight, your first changes may result simply in weight maintenance. Compared to weight gain, this is progress. Once your weight is steady, then you can focus on making further changes for weight loss.

2. TO CHANGE YOUR CURRENT RESULTS, YOU NEED TO CHANGE YOUR CURRENT HABITS, GRADUALLY:

Make small changes to your current habits focused on sustainability, rather than speed. Losing thirty pounds in eight weeks is useless if you gain forty pounds back over the following six months. Sustained change, no matter how fast, is the key to avoiding yo-yo dieting or buying yet another weight loss book that ends up as a paperweight (consider how many people who own three, five, or ten of these books yet are still overweight). The best pound lost or disease fought is the one that never comes back.

3. HABITS = CONSISTENT ACTION:

The hardest time to stick with changes is during the first few weeks. Just as a child gradually grows to become an independent person, our actions mature over time into permanent habits. The problem is that new actions are often replacing older, established, less healthy routines. And our body likes its comfort zone and status quo, so breaking old habits can be difficult. To combat this resistance, you must aim to use all of your available resources to turn the small changes from new actions into permanent, healthy habits.

4. OUR ACTIONS (AND HABITS AND RESULTS) ARE ALWAYS CHANGING BASED ON OUR THOUGHTS, CHOICES AND ENVIRONMENTS:

As life changes, so do our environments, thoughts and choices. Many situations can impact how you feel and what choices you make on a daily or weekly basis: skipping lunch due to a busy day at work can result in overeating at night. Moving due to a new job can mean losing sources of support and encouragement. The "irresistible" or "deserved" brownie after a long day of work or mindless munching of chips at your desk can sabotage your positive efforts. Keeping less healthy foods at home for the kids could mean you end up eating most of it. Maintaining habits and results is often a lifelong process that involves building a relationship between your brain and your body, *despite* changing environments and circumstances. The only thing constant in life is change—and how we respond to that change is what ultimately dictates our success.

This book reflects my experiences at gyms, hospitals, nursing facilities and in the community, working with people in their pursuit to change their weight and live healthier lives. Whenever people tell me that they have successfully made a significant, *long-term* change in their weight, fitness or health (over the course of years, not just months), I've made it a point to ask them how they did it, what allowed them to maintain their results and what tips they have for someone trying to do the same. After a while, I noticed that all of the people tended to have similar backgrounds and tips:

- They made changes both to their eating habits and their physical activity levels.
- The changes were typically small and gradual, but consistent and permanent.
- The changes were hard at first, but became easier over time.
- Results came slowly but were long-lasting.
- Setbacks and plateaus always appeared, but the people did not give up. Instead, they recognized the problem, found ways to resolve the issue as quickly as possible and got back on track.
- They believed that the process never ends, and expected to encounter new roadblocks and challenges to contend with and conquer.
- Rather than viewing setbacks as signs of failure, these people saw them as feedback. Adjusting and learning to grow from challenges is one of the biggest keys to long-term, permanent success.

This book and the Easy Eight Habits will create a framework of success for you based on honest assessment, small changes that can yield sustainable results, building support systems to convert new actions to permanent habits and empowering you to maintain your results no matter what life throws your way. But before we delve into these methods and concepts, I want to show you how this book stands apart from most of the standard diet and fitness books out there.

CHAPTER 2

DEATH OF THE DIET – THE ANTI-DIET BOOK

I'm not very happy about the state of affairs in the current diet and fitness book market. It seems that every week another fad diet emerges (eat grapefruits for breakfast, cabbage for lunch, a sensible dinner and only eat gluten on the third Tuesday of the month!) or extremely strict meal plan (no sugar, no alcohol, no meat, no breathing…) that typically leads to unsustainable results. The frustration of seeing so many people try book, after book, after plan, after book led me to conclude that the current model is just not working. How can someone own ten diet books and still be overweight? Something needs to change, and *Death of the Diet*, a book focused on changing long-term habits, is the answer.

DEATH OF THE DIET IS NOT A LOSE WEIGHT FAST SCHEME OR CRASH DIET

Let's say your child (or the child of someone close to you) is just starting to learn how to swim. Which teaching method do you think is better?

1. Give the child "floaties" or support him in the shallow end as he learns to kick his legs and paddle his arms in the water.

2. Toss the kid into the pool and tell him, "Kick your legs and paddle your arms! You can do it! Don't stop!"

I hope most of you chose option #1. This may sound like a ridiculous example, but option #2 is what crash diet plans are. Think about it for a minute. You know you want to make a change to live healthier (or in the case of the child, swim) but rather than make a few small changes (i.e. eating a few more veggies, walking a couple more times per week), you decide to cut out all sugar and red meat, exercise four days a week and take vitamins, fish oil and the latest supplements…just for good measure.

You throw yourself "into the pool" without floaties or support, and you wait to see if you sink or swim. Will you get results from those eating and exercise changes I mentioned? Sure you will! That's when you're kicking your legs and paddling your arms as hard as you can to stay afloat. But how long can you keep your head above water if you don't know how to swim? Forever? In the end, whatever results you achieve you must be able to maintain—through knowledge, action and experience—just like that child building solid swimming techniques step by step.

The problem is that most people with the "quick fix" mindset think that they can drink some green juices for two weeks, get the results they want and then go back to their previous habits without their body reverting to its original state. We are the results of our habits and actions. So if we go back to our *old* habits and actions…what do you think will happen to our new body? To maintain some results, some of those 10,000 changes you made during the crash diet need to stick. Otherwise you will be back to where you started and sometimes worse, since crash diets tend to create an even slower metabolism than before the diet. This is because we lose the source of our calorie- and fat-burning potential: our lean body mass, like muscle and bone.

Another symptom of the quick-fix mindset: it's not progress or a success unless the results are extreme and fast. Would you be happy if I told you that you would lose ten pounds in six months by making just a few small changes to your eating habits and physical activity? Some people would be thrilled, while others would say, "Well, that doesn't sound like much." Unfortunately, the media we see every day – The Biggest Loser, advertisements and the news at 11 – only highlights the sensational stories…because that's what's sexy and what sells. No one likes to hear about the person who ate a bit less at meals, ate more fruits and veggies, walked more and lost 50 pounds in two years and has kept it off for five years. We want to see or read about the person who had a life-changing event, completely overhauled her diet overnight, started working out five days a week, made a bet with her cardiologist, fought through knee pain and just lost 100 pounds in six months.

Unfortunately, the *speed* of weight loss has no impact on the *permanency* of weight loss. I recently read an advertised testimonial about a "doctor supervised" eating regimen. A participant described feeling defeated because she only lost about ten pounds after six months of making changes on her own. So she turned to the advertised program and lost *42 pounds in eight weeks*! But of course this program never followed up with her two, five or ten years later, because no company wants to be responsible for a person's habits years after finishing their program. Well, the program in this book is with you for the long term.

It's easy to make drastic changes for a short time, but eventually the body and mind push back. For every ten people you see advertised as losing forty pounds in eight weeks, odds are there's another ninety who did not get anywhere or lost forty pounds and then regained fifty. But the fad diet companies don't advertise that. They just say on their advertisements with extreme examples: "Results not typical."

So what are typical results? Research shows that weight regain does occur after most "diet" programs, even clinical ones. But, those people who have healthy eating and physical activity strategies in place that allow them to maintain weight loss for at least two years have a *much greater* chance of maintaining long-term weight loss. And these are the people we can learn from. In fact, there's a whole database devoted to the "un-sexy," yet very successful people who've maintained long-term weight loss: the National Weight Control Registry.

Now think again about the woman in the advertisement: would you rather lose ten pounds in six months if you knew that you only had a small chance of ever gaining those ten pounds back, or forty-two pounds in eight weeks if you knew that you had a significant chance of gaining those pounds back (and possibly more)? If your answer is still that you prefer losing forty-two pounds in eight weeks, then this book may not be right for you.

If you care about permanent results, you may need to reframe your idea of success. Every healthy decision made, every pound lost, each temptation averted, every mistake learned from…is success. If your ultimate goal is to lose fifty pounds, try losing ten pounds first by making some small changes. Then maintain that new weight for a month or two before trying to lose more weight. If you can keep that weight off, then those new eating and physical activity actions have likely become your permanent eating and activity habits. This will not only give you the confidence to make and maintain future changes, but will also make those changes easier to perform.

DEATH OF THE DIET IS NOT A RIGID, COOKIE-CUTTER MEAL AND WORKOUT PLAN

When people find out that I am a Registered Dietitian, nutritionist and personal trainer, they sometimes ask me to write a quick meal or workout "plan" that they can follow on their own to lose weight, improve their health or fitness, etc. All the while assuming they will automatically know how to correctly perform all of the exercises I list or how to integrate all of the new foods that I recommend into their lives and schedules.

If I said, "To lose weight, you must eat six small meals a day and cut all carbs from your diet except fruits and vegetables," would you lose weight? Probably. But are you willing to go the rest of your life eating every three hours while never having a piece of bread or pasta? If you aren't, then that cookie-cutter "plan" isn't right for you. And that's why I no longer write plans unless I spend a significant amount of time creating it with my client (in fact, they usually make the plan and I advise or give feedback). You can get a meal or workout plan anywhere—and you don't need to spend tons of money on it. Open a fitness or health magazine. Open any diet or workout book—I'm sure a few new ones have been published this year!

The problem is people are looking for that mythical magic bullet to solve their weight and health issues. That's why Americans spend tons of money on diet pills, medications, fad diets and workout plans, to the tune of $60 billion dollars per year. These magic bullet seekers start the latest fad diet or exercise plans thinking: "this plan will surely make the difference this time!" Yet they rarely consider the source of the information, their own preferences and whether they actually *can* or *want to* sustain these changes for the long haul – new habits like working out five days a week, eating no refined flour or sugar, etc.

All we're doing is temporarily treating the symptoms – our poor eating and activity habits – without addressing the source of the issue: our lifestyle and preferences. We follow others' temporary solutions blindly, without looking in the one place where our permanent solutions reside: ourselves. Unfortunately, listening to others without listening to *yourself* can lead to a number of issues including yo-yo dieting, injury and lots of frustration.

But we continue to follow these programs, see some results, fall off the wagon and gain all the weight back (or lose the weight if you are trying to gain). Then we start the next diet or workout plan thinking "this time it's different" when in fact nothing about our relationship with food or physical activity has truly changed. Does simply having a bunch of words on a page staring you in the face lead to permanent change? Think about how many weight loss, nutrition or fitness books you own and whether you are currently at your desired health or weight. The last thing this world needs is another diet or meal plan.

So what needs to change? As difficult as it may be to accept initially, we must change ourselves and our perception of what it means to "be healthy" or "fit" or "happy." Ask yourself: How will your health, fitness or weight (and ultimately your eating, physical activity and lifestyle habits) help you live the life you *want* to live? Do you want to avoid a family disease? Do you want to increase athletic performance? Do you want to go up stairs without getting winded? Do you want to see your kids get married and play with your grandkids? Ultimately, these answers are unique to each person. And with unique answers come unique solutions. So, any diet or exercise "expert" that offers you a one-size-fits-all approach with "results not typical" is selling you an approach that works for only one person...that expert.

I'm going to be totally upfront with you: I'm not psychic. If I was, you'd find me at the casino or racetrack. I don't know your daily schedule, your priorities, commitments, lifestyle, preferences and your reactions to stress and future life changes. So I'm not going to pretend I do. Giving you a highly-structured meal and workout plan through a book implies that I know you and all of the different things that you're dealing with in your life. Instead, I want to provide you with the framework, ideas and guidance needed for you to motivate and lead yourself to the solutions that work best for you. As I always tell my clients, two experts are involved in this process: I may be the expert in nutrition and fitness, but you are the expert in your own life.

SO WHAT IS DEATH OF THE DIET AND THE EASY EIGHT HABITS? – A COLLABORATION BETWEEN TWO EXPERTS: ME AND YOU

Though I'm not psychic, if you're reading this book I'm going to assume a few things (and if I'm wrong, please do tell me...my contact information is listed at the end of the book):

1. *You are not satisfied with your current health, fitness or weight results* – If you were satisfied, then you wouldn't need to make changes and you wouldn't need this book. Therefore, you acknowledge you are willing to change at least some of your current eating and physical activity habits.

2. *Most of the previous diet or workout plans you've read have not led to a long-term solution for you* – All too often, diet and exercise programs jump straight into *what* you need to do to lose weight or get fit, but they don't take the time to ask *why* you would be willing to give up carbs after 2 PM every day, start eating dairy and meat at each meal and go to the gym to immediately start doing lunges, squats, kettlebells and sprint intervals...even if you are a vegetarian who hasn't lifted a

weight in the past three years! Whether they were crash diets, juice cleanses or workouts of the week, results from these programs may have been fast, but not *permanent.*

3. ***You probably have an idea of what does and does not work for you based on your previous health, fitness or weight change experiences*** – Certain nutrition tips and strategies worked for your lifestyle and schedule while others didn't. You learned that you are good at and prefer certain types of physical activity. You know that some ideas or advice may not be right for your current health or medical status (for example, if you have injuries). You can maximize your chances for success by referring to these experiences and embracing your previous successes.

4. ***You accept that you haven't been able to guide yourself to your right solution on your own and are looking for some guidance to get there*** – When I talk to people about nutrition counseling, some will say, "I don't need nutrition advice or coaching, I know what to do and how to eat healthy. Fruits and vegetables, less soda and fried foods, yada, yada, yada. I just don't want to do it (or my schedule doesn't allow me to do it)." And the last sentence explains the exact reason why they need someone to help. Knowing is just half the battle…it's about taking consistent action. In other words, it's not just about *what* to do, but also *how* and *why*!

If knowledge were all it took for people to be healthy and fit, then nearly 70% of America wouldn't be overweight or obese and I would be out of a job (or at least working much less). But as we've all learned, knowing what to do doesn't automatically translate into doing it. Everyone needs to find their own motivation and desire to take action on their knowledge, while learning from their mistakes. This is how healthy actions become healthy habits that support the lives we all want to live.

In research, getting people to turn knowledge into action is called "bridging the attitude-behavior gap." To help people bridge this gap, many clinical diet and exercise programs include a behavior-related intervention such as regular meetings with a mental health, nutrition or fitness professional. Interestingly, behavioral-based interventions almost always have better results than knowledge, handouts or pills alone. Studies have shown that both in-person and virtual (email or phone) behavior intervention programs are significantly more effective in getting results. Why? Because ultimately your behavior, actions and habits dictate your results. And changing behavior requires taking an objective look at your current situation and developing the motivation to change.

This is where another person's perspective is extremely useful. All too often we get stuck in our own heads and get bogged down in worry, indecision or even fear of change or failure. Meeting with a fitness or nutrition professional, or reading a book focused on making small changes, can provide the right jolt needed to get you to start venturing outside the comfort zone of your current routines without feeling overwhelmed by an unrealistic plan.

And that's what this book is for: to coach you through the process of looking outside the box of your current lifestyle, and get you to achieve permanent results. Throughout the book you'll be reviewing your current eating and physical activity habits and determining what changes you can make consistently to start on the path towards getting those results. But most importantly, through this process you will come to the realization that:

1. You know most of the answers to your own problems, you are just not aware of them yet.

2. The best form of advice you can get from a nutrition or fitness expert is coaching (motivation and accountability), guidance (learning how to prepare certain foods or perform certain exercises) and useful ideas… not a mandated plan.

3. The solutions that you develop yourself, with the guidance of an expert, will be the ones you are most likely to stick with…because they are *your* solutions! Not a diet or fitness plan written by someone who claims to know your body and your life without ever having met you!

Within Death of the Diet you will probably see some recommendations similar to those presented in other diet or workout books. But unlike in those books, there are no rules or edicts. Instead, think of these recommendations as examples or a springboard for your own ideas. I want to give you the guidance and control to choose what changes work best for you, and help you create a plan to implement them. While I can provide support, guidance and ideas for you, you must ultimately be willing to take charge and change yourself.

Imagine you're driving down the road of life. You're the driver. I'm in the passenger seat giving support and directions. Let's buckle up!

CHAPTER 3

WHY CHANGE?

There's a saying that when your "why" is big enough, the "what" and the "how" will become clear. For now, don't worry about how you are going to change to lose your weight or improve your health, just focus on *why* you want to make these changes in the first place. Imagine yourself in six to twelve months having accomplished your fitness, wellness or health goals. What will you look like? How will you feel? What will be different about your daily routine?

Looking better, feeling stronger and having more energy are all fine reasons, but are they the true, underlying reason *why* you want to change? Or is there something more?

- Why do you want to look better? For yourself? For your significant other? For your job?

- Why do you want to have more energy? To play with your kids after work? To be able to play the sports you used to enjoy?

- Why do you want to be healthier? To be able to see your kids grow up to adulthood? To see your grandchildren? Because you don't want to end up like your mother, father, relative or friend?

Now you've started getting to the deeper meanings. Take it a step further:

ask yourself why you chose those reasons? Do you want to look better for your spouse because you feel insecure that she might no longer find you attractive? Do you want to have more energy to play with your kids because you want them to see you as an active, healthy role model? Do you want to have more energy to play with your kids because you want them to see you as an active, healthy role model? Do you worry that you are limiting your career progress due to how you look or how you feel? At this point, thinking about Why starts to get uncomfortable—and that's the goal!

The true Whys hit you in the gut, pun intended. They feel uncomfortable. They may even make you cry. Those are your true desires to change. And knowing your Whys is the first step to making permanent changes in your habits, health, weight and life.

Note: I started capitalizing the W in why. Moving forward, when you see the terms "Why" or "Whys," it is referring to your personal reasons for making positive changes to your health, fitness or weight.

FLIPPING THE SWITCH

Flipping the switch means turning on a "light bulb" inside of you that shifts your focus and priorities to your health, fitness, weight and well-being. Others call it an "a-ha" moment. Once you've flipped the switch, there's no turning back. You're determined to eat, move and live better to achieve the results you want, come hell or high water. You accept that long-term results do not happen overnight. Instead, they come by undertaking consistent action. For many who struggle with their health or weight, flipping the switch is a race against time. Eventually our health, or lack thereof, catches up to us.

Some of the people I've worked with define a very particular event or a-ha moment in their life that made them decide to change their eating and physical activity habits for the better. For example, they may have watched the scale tip above a certain number, received an unwelcome diagnosis from their doctor, could not fit into a seat on the train or at a restaurant, were taunted or stared at by strangers or saw a loved one pass away from diabetes, heart disease or obesity. These are the people who come in eating pizza and wings one day and then grilled chicken, salads and brown rice the next.

Of course, these people indulge on occasion, and they enjoy their indulgences. But afterwards they are focused on returning to their healthy habits as soon as possible, because they now know *Why* they want to be healthier. To live to see their kids grow up. To no longer be "that fat guy." They are able to strike a balance between their eating habits, physical activity and their quality of life. It seems like something happened to them overnight. And indeed, the *process* of change can start in an instant…the instant you choose to take action.

But not all of us will have such a radical change. In fact, most do not. Usually we start implementing little changes over time, seeing what works and what doesn't. In a lot of ways, it's like flipping on a switch with a dimmer option. We turn up the intensity gradually based on our current habits, situations and results. We build confidence as we accomplish and sustain our successes, bit by bit. And we can adjust it over time. But in the end, our switch is on and there's no turning back.

Unfortunately, many of the events that I describe above do not get people to change. It may make them feel bad or feel like they *want* to change…but they still choose to prioritize their current habits over their health. No one else can make you flip the switch; this chapter of asking, "Why change," however, will help you to flip the switch within yourself and start taking action.

ASK YOURSELF: WHY? WHY? WHY?

Close your eyes and imagine yourself in six to twelve months. On a piece of paper or the space provided on the next page, write down one to three weight, fitness or health results that you want to accomplish based on making positive changes to your eating and/or physical activity habits. Some common results include losing weight, being more toned or having more energy—but of course, what matters here is what's important to you. Then, rank how motivating each of them is to you from zero (no motivation to change) to ten (the largest motivating factor in my life, above *all* other commitments).

DESIRED HEALTH, FITNESS OR WEIGHT RESULTS – YOUR WHY	MOTIVATION TO CHANGE (0 TO 10)
1.	
2.	
3.	

Now look at each result again and ask yourself: "Why do I want to achieve these changes? How will achieving this allow me to live a better life or do things I'm currently not able to do?" Dig deep…usually our initial desires have deeper reasons. Weight loss, strength, energy, toning are means to an end—what's your end? What are you going to use this new-found slimmer weight, stronger body, greater energy for? That's your Why.

If you find a deeper Why than the result you initially listed, draw an arrow at the end of the original reason and write down the new one. Rate the motivation gained from this new reason. It will likely be higher than the original reason. Repeat this process for all of your desired health, fitness or weight results so each one has tangible life improvements associated with it. These are your true Whys. You can use the space provided on the next page or if you used a piece of paper, write them next to the original Whys.

If I initially decided I wanted to lose 30 pounds, here are two examples of potential deeper Whys:

- I want to lose 30 pounds (Motivation: 4) → I no longer want to get winded doing everyday activities like going up stairs and walking a few blocks. (Motivation: 7)

- I want to lose 30 pounds (Motivation: 4) → I want to look great in all of my old clothes that no longer fit (a particular dress or pants size?) (Motivation: 6) → I want to feel confident in myself and my body. (Motivation: 8)

ORIGINAL DESIRED WEIGHT, HEALTH OR FITNESS RESULT AND MOTIVATION SCORE	DEEPER REASON FOR DESIRED WEIGHT, HEALTH OR FITNESS RESULT AND UPDATED MOTIVATION SCORE
1. ▶	
2. ▶	
3. ▶	

If you're having trouble with this activity, read the next section on the Seven Dimensions of Wellness. Spend a couple minutes sitting and thinking about each dimension of wellness and how your health, fitness or weight can impact it. Then come back and give this activity another whirl.

IDEAS FOR DEFINING LIFE IMPROVEMENTS: ANSPAUGH'S SEVEN DIMENSIONS OF WELLNESS

While "wellness" has been a popular term used in the health and fitness fields, many people (myself included) find it vague. Does it mean happy? Does it mean fit? Does it mean low stress? Someone please explain! And thankfully, someone did. David Anspaugh and other researchers looked to make the idea of wellness a bit more concrete. As a result, they developed the "Seven Dimensions of Wellness," which provides a great insight into where we can derive satisfaction from life.

Adapted from a fantastic newsletter provided by Franklin Pierce University:

> "Wellness is a lifelong process of change and growth that is largely determined by the decisions you make about how to live your life. The dimensions of wellness interact continuously, influencing and being influenced by one another. Individually and collectively, the wellness dimensions are associated with quality and quantity of life."

In other words, the more we can maximize our happiness within each dimension of wellness, the happier our overall lives will be. And since our eating and physical activity habits can influence everything from our weight to our mood, energy and health, they can impact many of these dimensions of wellness simultaneously...for better or worse. Take a look at the description of each dimension of wellness below and consider how achieving your health, fitness or weight results will maximize your quality of life.

Social Happiness – Do you want to change any ways that you interact with your significant other, family, friends or even co-workers? Do you feel that your health, fitness or weight is keeping you from meeting the person of your dreams? Do you feel you have someone to turn to when you have troubles or challenges? Do you have a support network of caring friends and/or family members? Achieving relationships like these could be one of your Whys.

Emotional Happiness – How do you want to feel about yourself, others or life? How do you feel about your relationship with food and physical activity? Do you no longer want emotions to dictate your eating and physical activity habits? Do you want to have a more positive outlook on life? Do you want to feel more capable dealing with the challenges life throws at you? Do you want to have the confidence and self-esteem to know that you can bounce back from setbacks? Maintaining emotional wellness requires monitoring and exploring your thoughts or feelings, identifying obstacles to emotional well-being and finding constructive solutions to emotional problems. Your Whys might include the ability to do some of these activities of emotional happiness.

Occupational Happiness – Consider career and financial satisfaction as well as work/life balance. Does your current job give you the time to be active? Does your workplace promote healthier choices? Can making changes in your health, fitness or weight give you the confidence to ask for that raise or make a long-awaited career change? Do you feel that your employer makes decisions in your best interest? Maybe your Whys include taking control of your career.

Intellectual Happiness – Do you want to feel that your brain is actually guiding your body rather than just renting the space above your neck? Do you want to reclaim the feeling of what it's like to be hungry and satisfied rather than starving and stuffed? Do you want to be confident in the knowledge that the movements and activities you do on a regular basis are promoting health and strength rather than chronic discomfort and potential injuries? Do you want to be open to new ideas, have the capacity to question, or be motivated to master new skills? How about developing a better sense of humor? Your Whys might involve strengthening your mind-body connection, and bringing new energy to your intellect along with your body.

Physical Happiness – Do you want to reduce your risk for disease or complications? Do you want to control your blood sugar? Do you want to finally be able to have a child (yes, obesity is a factor in fertility)? Do you want to feel better "in your own skin?" Remember, weight is just a number; it does not dictate how we *feel* at that weight. And feelings last a lot longer than a number, so focus on those instead. Your Whys could include putting you and your body on the "same team," knowing that you're taking care of it so that it will sustain you for many years to come.

Spiritual Happiness – This is in reference to your personal beliefs, which may or may not include a higher power. What do you believe about yourself, your values and your principles? What is important to you and worth fighting for? This is your internal compass that guides you through the decisions you make in life and gives your actions meaning and purpose, especially during difficult times. Perhaps your Whys involve living more in tune with this internal compass.

Environmental Happiness – Think about how you want to interact with the natural world around you. Do you want to change your impact on air or water quality? Do you want to move towards sustainable agriculture or help your local farmers? Do you want to do your part to leave a safe and pleasant environment for your children and grandchildren? Your Whys may involve recognizing and embracing your role in the natural world.

Other – Any other driving force for accomplishing your Why that you feel is not represented by the other aspects of wellness listed above.

You do not need to have one Why for each of the seven aspects of wellness listed above. These examples are designed to get you thinking about your true, motivating desires. It's generally worth having at least one life improvement associated with a desired health, fitness or weight result, but more or less is fine. In the end, the most important thing is that these life improvements become your deeper reasons for change…your Whys.

EXAMPLES OF WHYS

If your initial desired result was to "lose weight" or "lose 30 pounds," some deeper reasons (Whys) for that weight loss could be:

- "I don't want to get winded trying to do every day activities like climbing stairs and walking a few blocks."
- "I don't want to feel like 'the fat guy/friend/relative' anymore."
- "I want people at work to respect me and acknowledge me for who I am, not how I look."
- "I want to look sexy and feel confident wearing that red dress."
- "I don't want to be self-conscious when taking off my shirt at the beach."

These statements create images and motivations that can inspire change much more than "losing 30 pounds." Why? Because they link weight loss with actual feelings and events that happen regularly in your life – rather than just seeing a number change on a scale every two weeks. If you can find a concrete feeling or event associated with making a change, then you are much more likely to take action on it. For all of your Whys, you need to *find the feeling*.

Also, be sure that your Whys are framed *positively*. Our mind responds much better to positive thoughts and results, so do your best to take any negative-based Whys and turn them around. For example, we can change some of the previous examples to:

- "I want to be able to bound up the stairs two at a time and feel great."
- "I want to be able to walk around all day and feel energetic."
- "I want my strengths and abilities to be obvious to others."
- "I want to feel confident when I take my shirt off at the beach."

Here are a few more life-changing Whys I have heard from clients:

- I want to lose weight so I can get pregnant and start my family.

- I want to lose weight so I can live pain-free and no longer be impacted by the arthritis in my knees.

- I want to lose weight so I can love myself and allow others to love me for who I am.

- I want to have more energy so I can be an active participant in my kids' lives rather than just lying around exhausted all of the time.

- I want to get stronger so I can keep my bones healthy to avoid having the osteoporosis that led to my mom breaking her hip in her sixties and not being able to move for months.

- I want to live better and lose weight to show that I am not a product of my genes. I will avoid getting the same disease (heart disease, diabetes, etc.) that has stricken or killed my family.

- I want to get stronger and have more energy so I can stop feeling like the world and my life is passing me by.

MY WHY

For me, flipping the switch started with two events: seeing the scale tip to the highest weight of my life while going through a difficult breakup. Yet as I started making changes and seeing results (results that I had gotten before but never managed to maintain), my Whys got deeper. I realized that I had always been insecure about my body, particularly the distribution of fat across my upper body, also known as "man boobs." I was the kid who always kept his shirt on at the pool and beach and was self-conscious about standing up straight. I was sick of that insecurity and it was time to let it go—feeling comfortable in my own body was my Why.

So over the course of ten months, I slowly, but steadily shed over thirty pounds and significantly increased my confidence in myself and my body. As a result, I began dating more than I ever had before (granted, it still wasn't a ton!) and was inspired to change careers to work with people taking the same journey. I changed my weight, but more importantly, I changed myself in the process.

KEEP YOUR WHYS WITH YOU TO STAY MOTIVATED

Your Whys need to *drive* you to make better choices, even when the deck is stacked against you—or to have the awareness and confidence to change the deck. A true Why is strong enough to get you out of bed at 6 AM (or into your gym clothes at 8 PM) to do your workout despite cold weather or long days. The real Whys will keep you *focused* so you can turn down the free cookies at work and instead eat the healthier snack you brought from home. Or you can decline the second piece of cake offered at a birthday party because you recognize that the first piece satisfied you. The real Whys will keep you *aware* that your longing for your favorite "comfort food" at the end of a stressful day is most likely related to emotion, not true hunger.

Once you feel that you've hit upon your most motivating and meaningful Whys, write them down on a couple of index cards or sticky notes, or type them on your computer or phone. Then place those cards or notes in places where you will see them every day and where you want to be motivated to make healthy decisions. You could keep them:

- On your night stand
- In your wallet or purse
- On your computer/screensaver at work

- In your car
- On your refrigerator
- Programmed as daily reminders in your phone

Take a minute to think about your Whys once or twice a day. When reviewing your Whys, imagine yourself as if you have already accomplished them. Try to hear, feel, describe and sense everything that would be occurring in your life when you've reached your Whys. Here are some of the best times when you could review them:

- First thing in the morning
- Right before bed

- During parts of the day when you have downtime, such as waiting in line
- At the end of the workday
- While exercising: during rest periods or cardio
- During the time of day when you know you have your biggest temptations or cravings

If you want to take it a step further, you could:

- Find an object that truly represents the feelings associated with your Whys, such as a particular piece of clothing or picture. Keep it with you or easily accessible, as a consistent, motivating reminder of your desire to change.
- Create a "mission accomplished" or success collage with pictures, meaningful words, images from magazines and any other media to represent your success. Make it your computer background. Print it out. Make a scrapbook. Do it old school on poster board. It all works! Use the different aspects of wellness (emotional, physical, social, etc.) as guides for choosing your images: What will you be eating? What will you be wearing? Who will you be surrounded by? What job will you have? Where will you live? What will be important to you?
- Record your Whys and listen to them in the morning, before bed or even on continuous playback overnight!

After spending some time clarifying your Whys on your own, find someone who believes in you and share your vision with them; it will help you in multiple ways. Saying your Whys out loud will strengthen your focus on *achieving* them and telling someone else will start the process of creating a supportive network. Also, telling others increases motivation and accountability because they will likely ask you how it's going in the future!

REVISING YOUR WHYS

As you go through your health, fitness and weight improvement journey, you may realize that the Whys you wrote down today are no longer the driving factors in your pursuit of change. Some potential reasons may include:

- You found a deeper Why.

- You achieved your first Why and are looking to set your sights on another one.

- You feel like you are losing motivation to make or maintain your positive, healthy changes.

These are all signs that your *desire* to improve has shifted, and it's time to re-think Why you are making these life-improving changes in the first place. Here are a set of steps you can take to review and potentially adjust your Whys. It should take about five to ten minutes, though it may take longer the first couple of times you do it:

- **Step 1:** Sit down in a quiet place with your current Whys and say them out loud three times. Pay attention to how each Why makes you feel.

- **Step 2:** Envision the Whys in your mind for a minute or two. Pay careful attention to any alternate thoughts or ideas that enter your mind during this time. If you feel like you may forget the ideas or thoughts, write them down and then go back to imagining your Whys.

- **Step 3:** Ask yourself if each of your current Whys still motivate you to continue the changes you have made to improve your health, fitness and weight. Don't just listen to your brain; listen to your heart and gut.

- **Step 4a:** If the answer to Step 3 is yes and you feel a renewed sense of inspiration, then you are still on the right path and may have just needed to reconnect with your Whys. This can happen if you're busy and dealing with many distractions (and as a result may not be reviewing your Whys daily).

- **Step 4b:** If the answer to Step 3 is no, use the activity from earlier in the chapter to identify new Whys. Anything that popped into your head while envisioning your current Whys is a good place to start.

Some examples:

- A person who already lost weight now re-orients to train for a 5K or to start playing a new sport.

- A person had been making changes to look better because she thinks it will increase her chances of a promotion. But she eventually decides that work should not play such a central role in her self-worth, so she chooses to improve her fitness for herself or her family instead.

Review your Whys at least every two to three months to make sure you feel like you're still on track. Your desired results and Whys may change as you learn more about yourself and start making some of the Easy Eight Habit changes. Above all, if you ever feel like you're losing motivation, re-examine your Whys, because they're the foundation from which all changes come.

CHAPTER 4

WHAT MAKES THE EASY EIGHT "EASY": CREATING SMALL, LONG-TERM CHANGES

As I hope I've already established, this is not a diet book. When I say "your diet," I'm referring to your usual eating habits, since that's the true, original definition of the word. Going "on a diet" is a temporary fix; changing your diet, or regular eating habits, is a solution. When people say they are on a diet, that usually translates to: "I am following a pre-determined set of rules that I do not enjoy doing, but will do anyway for a while until I lose some weight for an event or I just get tired or frustrated and give up." What happens after the event? What happens if you give up? Let's take a closer look at the statement above:

A pre-determined set of rules: Most diets require you to make a significant change in your eating routine, such as eliminating all carbs, only eating "raw" foods or eating cookies/grapefruit/meal bars/shakes for all of your meals until dinner.

...that I do not enjoy doing: Most people do not enjoy going on diets, especially ones that focus on restriction. This may be the reason why your co-worker or classmate is always pissed off...a diet may be to blame! Think about the last time you were on a diet. What was your energy level like? How did you

feel? Were you hungry? Were you happy?

On the flip side, some diets focus on only eating healthy foods (fruits, veggies, nuts, sprouted breads, etc.) all day, forsaking all other treats that you may want to have sometime between now and forever (meat, processed foods, chocolate cake, etc.). In theory that is a great diet, but the problem is maintaining it. If you can keep it up for a lifetime, then it's no longer a diet. It's your eating habits.

...until I lose some weight for an event or I just give up: We usually plan on diets ending, either by reaching our goal or by getting frustrated and giving up. Then what? Will you stay the same size, physique or weight after reverting to your old eating and physical activity habits? How did you get to your higher weight in the first place? By creating an endpoint to your diet, you are essentially admitting that the changes you have made are not sustainable, and therefore neither are the results you achieve. This is one of the key differences between a diet and eating habits: permanency.

Studies show that many kinds of diets, from low-carb to juicing, do lead to weight loss – but few people keep extreme diets like that up for long, so few keep that weight off for long. If you can't do it consistently, for years or a lifetime, then you will likely revert back to your old habits and old results. We need solutions that can be performed regularly.

FAST RESULTS ARE NOT ALWAYS THE BEST RESULTS

Think about the following facts:

1. Very quick weight loss tends to erode your precious lean body mass (muscle, bone, etc.) much faster than steady, consistent weight loss does. Yet lean mass is what burns the vast majority of your calories each day, while keeping you strong so you can stay active throughout your life. So losing too much lean body mass from a crash diet actually makes maintaining that weight loss even harder due to a slower metabolism and decreased strength. This issue is magnified if you are not staying active and performing resistance-based activities such as calisthenics or weight lifting.

2. And to keep those fast results, you also need to continue performing most of the actions you've started doing…consistently. Forever. Can you do it? If you're starving yourself on 800 calories a day, then probably not.

If you do something regularly, it stops being a diet and becomes your eating habits. Unfortunately for the vast majority of us, diets do not become eating habits…they become small "breaks" along the road of unhealthy eating and further weight gain. Perform this routine repeatedly and that is called "yo-yo dieting." That's how we go on four diets over five years and end up *gaining* 30 pounds in the end! And research indicates that chronic weight cycling may be associated with greater fat stores around our mid-section, which is tied to a number of chronic diseases such as hypertension and diabetes.

HOW HARD ARE YOU PUSHING THE SPRING?

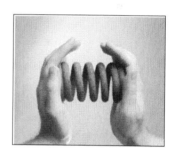

So why do crash diets and quick weight loss schemes never seem to work in the long run? We choose to go on temporary diets and binges of physical activity *without ever actually changing our underlying relationship with the food we eat or how we move our bodies.* How long can you continue to do something you don't want to do before you get frustrated, rebellious, cranky or injured?

It's like running full steam ahead into a spring against a wall. You will make quick progress using the momentum of your initial charge, but as time progresses, you start to feel an uneasy force pushing back on you. That's when you realize that you've pushed way too hard on the spring and you haven't had the time to build the knowledge and strength to produce enough effort to maintain the spring's position. So what happens? The force of the spring pushes back…hard. Then, do you get pushed back to where you started? Or, do you get thrown even further back into worse habits (such as binging) than when you started? That's why we can lose thirty pounds one year to gain back forty pounds over the next two years. And do it again three years later.

Why do we keep doing this to ourselves? It's because all diets *do* work, at least for a while. So we keep getting teased to run into that spring rather than learning what really makes the spring move – our eating and physical activity habits. Our body's response – that is, the spring's tension – is easier to manage under small, sustained pressure than when we've applied huge, uncontrolled efforts. Staying aware of this, we can take a few small steps to push against the spring and get a feeling for what level of pressure and changes are truly sustainable. Or we can feel which changes are just asking to throw us back to where we started. And the longer we stay at a certain level of pressure, the stronger we get and the easier it becomes to take another step. And finally, this time things *will* be different.

AN ACTIVITY FOR CHRONIC DIETERS OR THOSE FEELING "STUCK" IN THEIR CURRENT HABITS

If you've tried a bunch of diets in the past, do this activity: Divide a piece of paper into five separate columns. At the tops of the columns, write down the last five diets you were on. Then for each diet column, write down the following information:

- How long you were on the diet (specific dates work best, in chronological order).
- What the diet involved doing/restricting/changing.
- The results of the diet.
- How you felt during the diet.
- What caused the diet to end?
- What happened to your weight or physique over the six to twelve months following the end of the diet (assuming you didn't start a new diet)?
- What about the diet worked for you? Think about things you could see yourself doing again…for the long-term.

- What did not work for you in the diet, and potentially led to you ending the diet?

If you don't have a history of dieting but feel stuck in your current habits, despite wanting to make a change, think about and answer the following questions on a piece of paper:

- Was there a time when you were happy with your health, fitness or weight? Describe that time, and the habits you had then.

- How did you get into your current situation?

- What has changed between then and now? How did those changes create your current habits?

- Is there anything you used to do that you can start doing again?

- If you've never been happy with your health, weight or fitness, consider what you think you may need to feel or experience to know that you are breaking out of your current habits and making positive changes.

Using this information, you can likely get a sneak peek into which actions and Easy Eight Habits will be easiest for you to start with. In other words, if you know you like fruits and veggies, it might be easier to start adding in food to your diet rather than cutting things out. By adding those fruits and veggies to your meals and snacks, you will likely get fuller faster or be less famished at meals, so you will naturally eat less. And eating less results in fewer calories consumed, which typically means a slimmer waistline!

MOVE THE SPRING SLOWLY & PERMANENTLY WITH SMALL, LONG-TERM CHANGES

Let's think again about the spring from earlier in the chapter for a moment:

- What is the spring? It's our bodies' response to change.

- Why do we want to move the spring? To accomplish our Whys.

- What's moving the spring? Our actions and efforts to eat better and/ or move more.

- What force is pushing back on us via the spring? The resistance that our current preferences, lifestyle and schedule presents to our eating better or moving more. Our current comfort zone.

You want to move the spring, but you need to do so in a way that allows you to not only achieve, but maintain the progress you make. As you read earlier, making lots of quick changes is usually not a great option. Instead, a slower, steady force of positive change can get you gradual results that minimize the negative feelings of dieting, restricting or giving up other important aspects of your life. Remember, these eating and physical activity changes are designed to make your life better, not worse!

Building our strength to withstand the resistance of the spring comes from the following five approaches:

1.   MAKE SMALL CHANGES BASED ON YOUR CURRENT HABITS

You are performing your current habits for a reason. They are probably the "easiest" things for you to do based on your current schedule and priorities. They are the path of least resistance (think about the spring), the status quo, your comfort zone...insert any additional cliché here. But, these current habits are not getting you the results you want. So change needs to happen. However a huge, fast overhaul to your habits can create an unpleasant shock to your system – much like a frog does not want to be thrown into boiling water.

Frog lovers and animal activists please know that I harmed no frogs in the making of this paragraph. I recently heard how to cook a live frog, though I don't ever plan on doing it. However, I found the parallel to making small changes compelling. As I mentioned, if you try to throw the frog in boiling water, it will immediately hop out. It knows that the hot water is very different from its current environment and will reject it. However, if you place it in a pot of room temperature water, turn on the stove and then let the water get warmer over time, the frog will not sense the gradual increase in temperature until it's too late and frog soup's on. We are like the frog. We tend to rebel against big changes.

Similarly, subjecting yourself to huge changes in eating habits and physical activity routines means you would need to greatly alter your current habits to accommodate them. How accommodating is your schedule right now? Can you make the time to go from working out once a week to four times a week? Can you devote half of your Sunday every week to preparing your meals for the week? Are you ready to say bye-bye to all of your daily indulgences? Don't think about how you will feel about it next week. Instead, think about maintaining all those changes for the next year, or two or five. Makes you want to jump out of the water too!

And who knows if you actually need to make all of those changes to get the results you want. It's about working smarter, not harder. Since you know your current habits have created your current results, all you need to do to start making improvements to your results is to make one consistent, positive change to your habits. Maybe you would only need to work out one extra day, walk a bit more, sit a bit less and have a couple fewer desserts per week to get the results you want – all of which can fit into your schedule.

Honestly, you probably won't know the right combination of changes until you get there, so why not start in comfortable water and dial up the temperature slowly? Make one change, see how it goes and then adjust based on the results. Then make another change. You'll be much more likely to stick with future changes if you're comfortable with the current ones.

2.   FOCUS ON ONE CHANGE AT A TIME

Often you'll have lots of great ideas on how to make improvements to your eating and physical activity habits. But focus your efforts only on the ones that *maximize* your chances for long-term success based on your current situation. Here are a few reasons why focusing on only one small change at a time can be the best approach:

- Choosing one change to focus on avoids "analysis paralysis" where you get overwhelmed by so many options, you end up doing none!

- It lets you choose what you consider to be the easiest change first. Easy doesn't just mean simple, it means you can fit it into your current lifestyle and make a concerted, focused effort to achieve it. Early success builds confidence and creates momentum for future changes and success. If the change seems complex, you can make it even easier by breaking it down into individual actions and steps. More on this in Chapter 8.

- It lets you focus on the same change for at least three weeks before moving on to the next idea. Studies show it takes at least three to four weeks for new actions to become habits. If you try to move on too soon, it reduces your chances of any of the changes sticking.

- It increases the chance of success. According to John Berardi, founder of Precision Nutrition, you have about an 85% chance of making one change, a 33% chance of making two and a near 0% chance of making three or more changes at the same time.

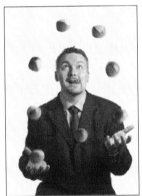

It's like trying to juggle (for juggling experts, pretend you have just started learning). Each ball is equal to one eating or physical activity change, such as "one more fruit or veggie," "one less soda" or "one more day of activity." It's pretty easy to juggle one ball. It's a bit challenging but doable for most to juggle two balls. But add a third or fourth ball and the vast majority of us start doing a crazy dance of "oh crap, don't let the ball fall." And it usually does fall, pretty fast.

Then do we continue to juggle the remaining balls, or do we just stay focused on that one dropped ball, call ourselves a "failure" and let the rest of the balls drop as we sit around eating junk food the rest of the week? That's the issue of crash dieting, making too many unsustainable changes. Why not get really good at juggling one ball and then two before jumping all the way to three?

3.   PRACTICE, PRACTICE, PRACTICE

Successful businessman Marshall Thurber once said, "Anything worth doing well is worth doing poorly at first." When you wanted to learn to play a sport, play an instrument or learn a language, did you get fed up the first time you missed a shot or made a mistake and say, "To hell with this, there's no way I'll ever be able to do it?" Or did you try again? And again? And finally you got pretty good at it, right?

Living healthfully, eating better and becoming active needs to be learned and practiced just like any other skill. There will probably be lingo you'll need to learn and some abilities you'll need to improve upon (opening cans, sautéing, portioning, using a treadmill, learning a new sport). If you've been active and eaten well in the past, you may just need to learn how to do it given your current schedule or demands. The only way to figure out which changes are best for you is to try, try and try some more. You will get better. It will get easier.

4.   GET SUPPORT & GUIDANCE

Effective support and guidance provides even more motivation and accountability to help you stick with your healthy changes until they become habits. The drive from support and guidance can come from others (external) or from within yourself (internal).

Classic forms of external support include having a workout buddy, a walking group at work, a friend or significant other that you can cook healthy meals with, a person you can talk to when you're having a stressful day, an accountability group like Weight Watchers, etc. These are people on the journey with you.

Getting external guidance means reaching out to others who have more experience or knowledge than you in a particular field. You can learn a lot via a book, guided practice, training, consultation or webinar.

Internal support is just as important: positive feelings and the belief that you can succeed in achieving your Whys. Having internal support means you embrace your strengths but recognize your limitations and take steps to address them (such as hiring a trainer or a nutrition coach for guidance or accountability, buying a book, etc.).

You will also learn to focus on your own thoughts and feelings for internal guidance on the next best step. The more you are attuned to your own needs, wants, demands, schedule and priorities, the better you can choose the changes and habits that are best for your life. The better the new actions fit, the more motivated you will be to perform them! And, the more in line the change is with what you truly want in life (your Whys), the more accountable you'll hold yourself to executing it.

Internal support and guidance is the most important set of skills to build for long-term success, because external support and guidance may come and go – friends move, nutrition or training sessions end, we change jobs. In the end we're always left with ourselves. *And no one can do your pushups or eat your fruits and veggies for you.* If you feel that your internal support and guidance skills are not as strong as you'd like them to be, consider investing in external guidance to build awareness of your Whys and to gain the knowledge and confidence to make positive changes to your eating and physical activity habits.

5.   TWEAK AND SUCCEED VIA EDUCATED TRIAL-AND-ERROR

Without a doubt, getting from where you are now (your current results) to where you want to be (your Whys and desired health, fitness or weight results) is a process. You may have an overnight shift in *thinking* about your eating and physical activity habits, but the *results* do not come overnight.

Making your health, fitness and weight loss changes easy to execute is the best way to convert your new actions into habits, and results. But unless you already know exactly how to integrate your proposed changes into your existing priorities, preferences and schedule, you're going to probably have to try a few things here and there to see what works for you. Some ideas will work and some won't. If a particular habit or change works, stick with it. And be sensitive to what's working; if your old habits had you gaining weight, then any habit changes that lead to weight maintenance is *progress*.

Keep in mind, though, that you're not going into this process blindly. Your priorities, preferences and schedule can also provide insights into what options are better than others. If you have a demanding work schedule, you may know that increasing walking or improving your eating habits could be a better first change than increasing your workout frequency. This is why I call it *educated* trial-and-error.

With trial-and-error, of course, comes error. Don't beat yourself up about a wrong decision. Accept it, learn from it and then change course. In fact, during this process you should expect to run into speed bumps – it shows you're making progress. One immutable fact is that **there is no such thing as failure, only feedback**™. Feedback includes learning from mistakes and becoming aware of what does and does not work for you. The one thing *not* to do is continue doing the same thing over and over and expect different results. That's Albert Einstein's definition of insanity.

Making changes in your health or weight is a blend of science and art. While all science works in theory (i.e. eat fewer calories than you burn and you'll lose weight), the true challenge comes in the art of taking consistent action on the science, day after day, year after year in your real life. It takes inspiration and creative thinking to shake up a familiar routine and introduce new patterns of behavior. This book aims to provide you insights and ideas for both the art and science.

Once you choose a science-based Easy Eight Habit to change in Chapter 7, you'll read some useful tips for taking action on that Habit. Then the following chapters provide you with guidance about translating those actions into long-term habits. Planning and strategizing is covered in Chapter 8, and learning to adjust based on feedback from your body, thoughts, lifestyle and results will be discussed in Chapter 9.

Ultimately as you progress in your journey of making changes, your desires and Whys serve as your compass, your "North Star." As long as you keep referring to your compass and adjusting your approach with the aim of progressing toward your Whys, then there's ultimately no stopping you from getting there…and staying there.

DEMYSTIFYING WILLPOWER: HOLDING THE SPRING IN PLACE

Many people view willpower as this magical ability that certain people have and others don't. They see it as a form of supreme control that we must exert on ourselves to "stay in line" and keep from going overboard. But if you ask a person who seems to have lots of willpower about their healthy eating and activity decisions, odds are they will tell you it's not hard at all. In fact, they may even say it's the easiest part of their day and they feel like something's missing when they don't eat well or make it to the gym on their scheduled days. The truth is, these people don't have better powers of self-denial than everyone else – they simply plan ahead so that they don't *need* to exert superhuman willpower.

They've found the right amount of pressure to exert on their spring to get the results they want, and they know how to keep it there. They enjoy eating healthy and being active—it makes them feel good. Do these people never miss a workout or always turn down dessert? Probably not. But rather than dwelling on it, they just focus on returning to their healthy habits as quickly as possible. It's not about perfection, it's about persistence.

In actuality, "willpower" just boils down to motivation and choice. We choose to eat better or be more active because we are motivated to do it. Why?

1. Because we want to do it. (Motivation from our Whys)

2. Because we know we can do it. (One small change at a time)

3. Because we know how to do it. Or can learn how. Or can get better at it. (Practice, practice, practice, guidance, support and adjustment)

4. Because we value our commitment to doing it. (Accountability)

5. Because we enjoy how it feels and *like* doing it. (Feedback and Motivation from our successes)

Does anything in that list involve negative reinforcement such as guilt tripping (calling yourself a "fatty" or putting negative photos on your fridge) or restriction (no carbs or sugar...ever! If I eat a carb, I'm a loser! I've failed!)? One of the most amusing negative reinforcements I ever saw was a framed fake-inspirational photo of Dr. Phil saying, "You're fat! And I'm not going to sugarcoat it either, because you'd probably just eat that too." Funny, yes. Effective motivator, probably not.

In fact, those kinds of strategies tend to lead to resentment and relapse because no one likes to be yelled at, especially your emotional subconscious (more on the subconscious in the Epilogue). Genuine, long-lasting willpower results from having *positive* thoughts and feelings about the healthy choices you make and then taking the steps needed to ensure you consistently follow through on those choices until they become a habit.

This is the essence of willpower: It's *not* about having to stare down a free cookie when you are hungry. It's about having a *strategy* to make sure that you either are not around the free cookies, have a healthy, satisfying snack available to keep you from being hungry around that free cookie, or a plan to eat and enjoy one cookie as a part of your daily eating routine. Nor is it about starving all day while traveling to avoid airport food. It's about bringing your own meals or figuring out the healthy airport food options that will be available to you before you get there. And then practicing these strategies repeatedly until they become a part of you and you no longer have to think about them. You just do them.

AN EXAMPLE OF THE POWER OF SMALL CHANGES

Let's say you're maintaining your weight with your current eating habits and exercising once a week. But you want to significantly improve your weight and fitness levels over the next six months and are thinking about making small, sustainable changes. On average it takes four weeks for a new action to become a sustained habit. So, over six months you would be able to make about six Easy Eight Habit changes:

- *Month 1*: Increase 1000 steps per day / 10 blocks = 350 extra calories burned per week.

- *Month 2:* Increase produce intake by two veggies and two fruits per week = consuming an extra 175 calories per week, but getting full faster at meal time and leaving food over.

- *Month 3:* Decrease portion sizes at main meals during the week by 20% by using smaller plates, having a fruit or veggie snack from last month's changes when hungry = 1000 calories saved per week, which equals about 150 calories less per day, or just 50 calories less per meal if you're having three meals per day.

- *Month 4:* Increase physical activity by one 45-minute workout per week = 350 extra calories burned per week. Due to getting hungry from being more active, you start having a post-workout snack of a low-fat yogurt and a piece of fruit previously added to the rotation in Month 2, fueling your body for strength and recovery by consuming an extra 150 calories per week.

- *Month 5:* Start sitting one less hour per day = 210 extra calories burned per week.

- *Month 6:* Reduce two indulgences per week: one pint of beer and two cookies = 350 calories saved per week.

Let's add the numbers up. At the end of the six months, you are burning an extra 910 calories per week AND consuming 1025 fewer calories per week. One pound equals 3,500 calories. So based on the habits you've accumulated over those six months, you would be losing about half a pound a week, which is 26 pounds a year. Not to mention you're getting the health and fitness benefits from extra physical activity and more fruits and veggies!

To get these results, all you had to do over the course of six months was this:

- Increase working out from once to twice a week
- Walk ten more blocks per day, about eight to ten minutes
- Sit one less hour each day, either at home, at work or commuting
- Eat two more fruits and two more veggies each week
- Leave some food on your plate, or use smaller plates, at meal time
- Eat a post-workout snack
- Have one less beer and two less cookies each week

Sound doable?

CHAPTER 5

THE SOLUTION: UPFRONT & UNCENSORED

I'm going to do something totally radical that may allow you to get the results you want without reading the rest of this book. I'm going to give you the solution to improving your health, fitness or weight right now. Ready? Here it goes:

Health, Fitness or Weight Improvement =
Consistently [Eat Better + Move More, Safely]
...than you are doing right now

If the equation above did not create an epiphany or a huge light bulb to pop up above your head, do not be alarmed. Most people read it and think, "Great, I get it. Now how the hell am I going to do it?" That's what the rest of the book is for!

The Easy Eight Habits described in Chapter 7 focus on gradually improving that equation: eating better and moving more, safely. Within that chapter there are assessments you can use to determine your current habits. Once you've established a baseline for change, there are tips to make starting the Easy Eight Habits as easy and safe as possible. Finally, the last two chapters provide guidance on how to take *consistent* action, so you can translate the Easy Eight Habits into permanent results.

CHAPTER 6

THE EASY EIGHT APPROACH TO ACHIEVING PERMANENT HEALTH AND FITNESS

The Easy Eight approach follows five steps. You continue through the steps until you reach your desired health, fitness or weight results—and ultimately your Whys.

1. Choose an Easy Eight Habit that works best for your current lifestyle and preferences.

2. Establish your current baseline by using the chosen Easy Eight Habit's assessment.

3. Start making the recommended Easy Eight Habit changes based on your assessment. Adjust the recommendation as necessary to fit your lifestyle, schedule or preferences.

4. Focus only on that Easy Eight Habit until you are confident that it has become a permanent part of your life. *Note: Research shows it can take up to four weeks to establish a new habit.

5. Since new habits create new results, reassess your current results: are you happy with them? Have you achieved your Whys? If yes, stick with your current habits. If no, and you want more results, go back to #1 and choose another Easy Eight Habit to make changes to.

6. Having trouble with an Easy Eight Habit? Read Chapters 8 and 9 again. Review or revise your Whys. Then once again ask yourself if you are

happy with your current results. If yes, stick with your current habits. If no and you want more results, go back to #1 and choose a different Easy Eight Habit to work on.

WHEN IN DOUBT, GO WITH THE FLOW(CHART):

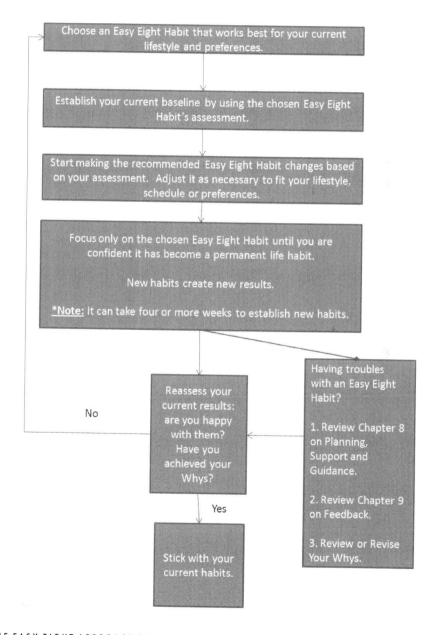

CHAPTER 7:

THE EASY EIGHT HABITS

At this point, you've probably been wondering what the heck the Easy Eight Habits are and why it's taken me so long to tell you about them. Well, the fact is these habits are pretty easy and self-explanatory...in theory. But something that's simple is not always easy. Just like "The Solution" in Chapter 5, it's not about the knowing...it's about the *doing*, consistently. Achieving your Whys will flow from your actions, which will flow from your mindset – so in keeping with this approach of starting from the mindset to make action easier, I broke each habit down into five components:

1. Name of the Habit
2. Rationale for the Habit: How it will help you reach your Whys
3. Assessment for the Habit to establish your baseline
4. Recommended changes to the Habit based on your assessment
5. Easy Habit Strategies: Tips to make the changes easier

HABIT 1: EAT MORE OFTEN

RATIONALE

Two common problems can be addressed by eating more frequently throughout the day. If your metabolism is stalled from chronic undereating (most women need to eat at least 1200 calories per day, and men need 1500 calories), eating more often can increase your daily calorie intake and kick-start your metabolism back into fat-burning mode. Or, spreading out your daily calorie intake more evenly over the course of the day, without changing the amount of calories you consume, will help you avoid energy crashes, reduce cravings and fuel your body from the moment you wake up until bedtime.

Here's a common spike-and-crash scenario: You eat breakfast around 7:30 AM, before you leave for work. You usually don't have lunch until about 1 PM, so you're kind of hungry around 10 or 11 AM. But you decide to just stick it out until lunch because it's not too far away. By lunch time you're starving, so you say yes to the first option your coworkers suggest, or eat whatever's available, even if it's not healthy. And you likely eat too much, too fast, because you're really hungry. This surge of food causes a post-lunch crash a couple of hours later, around 3 PM. And since dinner isn't until 7 PM, you need to get a "hit" of something, usually sugar or caffeine, to get you through the rest of the day. Or you just sluggishly wait it out until dinner, with the same cycle repeating itself: starving, overeat, crash.

Eventually you may stop eating breakfast because you're still so full from the huge dinner you ate the night before. Then you're down to two meals per day, with not-so-healthy snacks added in to prevent crashing midday. It's a vicious cycle that many people don't realize can become a significant hindrance to getting results; they think, "I'm not eating often, only two meals per day, so why am I not losing weight?"

The answer lies in how our bodies are designed to handle food. Research shows that people who eat less than three meals per day tend to have impaired appetite control. In other words, they may eat too much at meals or give into cravings more readily. This happens because after about four hours without food, the body begins to act like it's starving, even if it has have lots of fat available. Hormone levels change, hunger increases, focus decreases and more. If we continue to push off eating, our metabolism will start to slow down to make up for the lack of fuel coming through the system. But then when we do eat, our body drives us to make up for the period of "famine"…and then some.

If you don't eat often during the day, your body is probably starved for fuel most of the day and then gorged once or twice. However, the average person rarely needs more than 600-700 calories per meal. So, the excess calories from big meals are just stored as fat, rather than being used right away for energy. This isn't the best way to fuel your body, especially if you want to lose weight.

So how does increasing meal frequency, such as going from two meals to three meals or from three meals to three smaller meals and a snack, help this situation? Here are some benefits:

- *Planning:* Eating more frequently forces you to think about what you're eating, and usually involves planning, preparing or pre-purchasing meals or snacks to have with you during the day. The more you prepare, the more likely you are to stick with making a good decision when confronted with less healthy options, because you've already thought the situation through.

- *Home Cooking:* Eating more frequently often involves more home cooking or food preparation. Meals or snacks made at home tend to be more nutritious and lower in calories than food at restaurants, which usually has lots of added sugar, fat, salt and calories.

- *Stable Blood Sugar:* When you're fueled consistently throughout the day, your blood sugar is much more stable. When you have more stable blood sugar, you're less likely to be ravenously hungry. And most people make better decisions about food when they're not ravenously hungry – you can say no to the pizza and yes to the grilled chicken salad.

- *Cope With Stress Better:* Stable blood sugar leads to another great side effect: feeling more energized throughout the day. The better you feel, the better you can handle stress. The better you can handle stress, the less you want that ice cream to comfort you.

- *Less Cravings:* You'll avoid the vicious cycle of food cravings. Unhealthy food cravings often come from the blood sugar crashes that follow a big meal or sugary snack. These crashes can lead to unpleasant symptoms including headaches, fatigue, shakiness and even feeling ravenously hungry again. When someone feels like that, they tend to look for the nearest food regardless of whether it's healthy, overeat, get a sugar high and then crash again a few hours later. Wash, rinse, repeat.

- *Get More From Your Exercise:* Eating a healthy snack before and after a workout is great fuel for exercise. Studies show that better fueling leads to better workouts, more calories burned and better results – this is true for athletes at all levels.

- *Increasing Energy Levels:* You can "reset" your metabolism and energy levels. For example, if you find yourself ravenously hungry at dinner, not hungry in the morning and dragging during the day, try eating a little more throughout the day or having a mid-afternoon snack. You'll probably be less starving at dinnertime, so you end up having smaller dinners. And lo and behold you start getting hungry in the morning again...and your energy levels are boosted from fueling your entire day.

- *Lose Weight More Easily:* When you eat frequently, you're more likely to eat enough calories to maintain your metabolism – which promotes a leaner physique. Eating too few calories for your activity level can lead to a slowed metabolism, which makes fat loss harder because your body thinks it's starving, regardless of how much fat you're carrying.

ASSESSMENT

Track your eating habits using the Eating Habits Assessment form for three, four or seven days. The longer you track, the better. Include at least one weekend day, as eating habits are often different on the weekend. For this Habit, focus on your energy levels, hunger levels, time you ate and what you ate. Estimating how much you ate can be useful, but it's not vital. Feel free to use things like your phone camera or Pinterest to track your eating habits with pictures; just be sure to label the information you need, such as energy and hunger levels, time, etc.

RECOMMENDATION

Ideally, you'd eat a balanced meal or snack every three to four hours. Read through your eating habits assessment and highlight any large gaps in eating during the day – anything 6 hours or more. Aim to have a balanced meal or snack around the mid-point of one of those times. For example, imagine you eat lunch around noon and dinner at 7 PM; that's a 7 hour gap in eating. Aim to add a healthy mini-meal or snack around 3:30 PM, which is the mid-point between 12 PM and 7 PM. If you can schedule that extra meal or snack around a workout, even better! For more details on balanced meals and snacks, read the Easy Eight Habit strategies below.

Regardless of how often you're eating, the goal is to eat frequently enough so you're sitting down to a meal or snack when you're hungry, not ravenous, and finishing when you're satisfied, not stuffed. This loosely translates to keeping your hunger level between 3 and 7 (on a 1 = starving to 10 = stuffed scale).

EASY EIGHT HABIT #1 STRATEGIES

MAKE FOOD THAT FITS YOUR SCHEDULE

If another meal or snack doesn't fit easily into your daily routine, then you're much less likely to stick with adding it in the long run. So rather than trying to force a meal or snack into your schedule, figure out how you can craft one around your schedule. Lack of time and not having any healthy foods around tend to be the biggest issues. But a little bit of planning can go a long way.

When you're planning ahead and deciding what snack or small meal you'll have and when, consider the little bits of downtime you may have throughout the day: getting ready in the morning, right before work, between meetings, at your desk, right after work, commuting, or before or after workouts. Next, consider how long you have available. There's quite a difference between five, ten and thirty minutes; you may be able to wolf down a yogurt or piece of fruit and nuts in five minutes, while making a sandwich could take longer. Also consider what appliances you'll have handy; is there a fridge, microwave or can opener around to expand your food options?

The goal is to feel satisfied until your next meal without feeling stuffed in the moment.

SPLIT BIG MEALS INTO TWO

Remember the last time you got to a meal feeling starving? Did you eat faster than usual? Did you eat too much? Regardless of how hungry you feel, your body needs at least fifteen minutes to register the fact that you're full. You need to slow down to give your stomach a chance to catch up with your mouth. Otherwise you're likely eating more calories than your body actually needs.

Splitting big meals in half, whether you're eating a restaurant meal, takeout or something home-cooked, has two major benefits. First, it gives you a chance to find out whether half the meal was actually enough to make you full. Second, it's a convenient way to increase your meal frequency without eating more calories. The second half of your big lunch can become a mid-afternoon snack, or your leftovers from dinner can become tomorrow's lunch – you're eating all the calories in that big meal, just spread out more over time.

Cutting your meals into two doesn't mean that you should deprive yourself if you are truly hungry, though. The way to tell? Don't eat everything in 3.2 seconds as soon as you sit down at the table. Wait fifteen to twenty minutes after eating the first half of the meal to give your body a chance to respond. If you still feel hungry, then odds are you really are hungry and you should have a bit more. It's not about feeling restricted, it's about feeling in control of your eating decisions.

SCOPE OUT YOUR OPTIONS

Think about this: If you ate every three to four hours during the day, where would you eat? What type of food would be available to you? How could you prepare it? It's much easier to plan out a meal or snack when you know your options ahead of time.

People usually eat in one of six places: at home, at work, at someone else's home, on the run or while commuting, at a restaurant, or in airports or hotels while traveling. Knowing where you'll be eating can let you start planning whether you'll need to pack an extra snack for the day, preview a menu or even have a little bite to eat before you go somewhere.

AT HOME

Stock your pantry wisely – Imagine having both apples and Oreos in your home – which would you choose to eat? What if you only had the apple available? Are your pantry and fridge stocked with healthy options…or just snack foods? Don't even let those snack foods into your home. We prepare and eat what's around us, so upgrade the health of the foods you have in your home if you want to make the healthiest decision the easiest decision. Use the "Healthy Food Preference List" in the Appendix for ideas.

Think about tomorrow – If you're cutting up fresh fruits or vegetables tonight, prepare some extra now and put it in a plastic container for tomorrow. For example, if you're cutting up cantaloupe, you can dice up half of it rather than just a slice. You can bring some leftover melon to work the next day or have it around the house the next evening when you're in the mood for something sweet and healthy.

Make big batches – Want to prepare healthy meals at home in less time? Forget cooking for one; try cooking for five (days, that is)! A lot of the time spent cooking actually goes towards getting everything ready and then cleaning up – not cutting up and cooking an extra piece of chicken or carrot. Try whipping up a large batch of a recipe that you like, so you can eat it a few times that week for lunch or dinner. It only takes a few extra minutes of food prep, and you'll save tons of time and stress later in the week when you're busy or hungry. Divide your leftovers into individual containers and put them in the fridge or freezer as soon as you're done cooking, to keep the food safe from spoiling and to make it easy to eat a healthy portion size at the next meal. Then when you've had a long day at work later in the week, you can come home, reheat and enjoy dinner in seconds!

Pay a little extra for convenience – Life is always about time vs. money, isn't it? It's the same with prepared foods – there's the extra cost of the item, but there's also the time saved that you otherwise would have to spend making the food yourself. For example, paying three dollars for fifty cents' worth of chopped peppers and onions might not be worth the one minute of chopping you'll save. However, you may find value in paying an extra dollar or two for a big bag of prewashed and cut lettuce, which allows you to make a salad in half the time.

AT WORK

Buying food fresh – Do you pass by a grocery store, produce vendor or cafe on your way to work each day where you could pick up some healthy, whole food snacks? Or could you buy fresh food in large amounts and prepare them as future snacks at home over the weekend or the night before?

"Go-to" food joints – If you usually order food from the same couple of places, look through their menus for healthier options. Or take a walk around the area where you work to look for new places that may provide even better meals or snacks. Try one new place or new food each week. Soon you'll have healthy "go-to" places and meals so you'll be able to order without giving it much thought.

Access to a fridge – You can keep quick-and-easy meals fresh during the day until you need them. You can also have bulk foods on hand for several days, such as larger containers of fruit, veggies, yogurt, milk for cereal, hard boiled eggs, smoothies or grab-and-go snacks.

Access to a heat source – A toaster or microwave can open up a number of options. You can make a low-sodium frozen meal in minutes. Or you can cook a sweet potato in the microwave in about seven minutes by poking holes in the potato with a fork, heating on one side for about three minutes, turning it over and cooking it for another three or so until you can easily stick a fork in it (be careful, it's hot). Top the 'tater off with some yogurt and cinnamon for a fast, filling snack.

Access to utensils – You can bring silverware from home or keep some plastic utensils at your desk. You may also need a can opener.

AWAY FROM HOME

Eating on the run or while commuting –Sometimes your schedule just doesn't allow you to get a "proper" meal in—and that's fine. If your commute is long and begins after not eating for a few hours, treat that commute time as a meal or snack time too. Then you won't be starving by the time you get home or wherever you're headed. If you're running around all day, eat a series of mini-meals or snacks in place of a full meal. It's much better than waiting hours and hours for a meal, becoming ravenously hungry, overeating and then feeling sluggish the rest of the day or going to bed with a stuffed stomach. Having healthy snacks available where you are, of course, is the key (see the related strategy, *Always Have Something Healthy on Hand*, later in this section).

Eating at a restaurant or café – While this could be its own long chapter, here are some of the basics:

- Choose restaurants that offer healthy meals and side items, such as grilled and broiled meats, salads, vegetable-based entrées (not the mac and cheese), baked potatoes, fruits and steamed veggies on the side. Oh, and avoid buffets.

- Look for the words baked, roasted, grilled, broiled, steamed, cooked in its own juices, marinara or tomato sauce, choice or select cuts of meat, and broth- or tomato-based soups.

- Ask for salad dressings and dips on the side. Choose lower-calorie condiments like salsa, mustard and balsamic vinegar. Have them hold the mayo. If you do use a higher-calorie dressing or sauce, dip the fork into it before spearing a bite of food, rather than pouring it on top of the whole dish. You'll get a taste of the dressing in each bite, but eat much less in total.

- Ask for healthy substitutions, such as swapping French fries for a side salad or replacing hash browns with a side of fruit.

- Make two healthy appetizers – or one appetizer and a side salad – into a meal, or share entrées and desserts with a companion.

- Ask to have the bread or chips removed from the table.

- Eat slowly, and when you're done eating, immediately have the waiter wrap up leftovers or take the plate away. That way you won't be able to pick at it.

Travel and Vacation – Traveling is another challenging situation, especially if you do it on a regular basis. Consultants, speakers and others who travel often can benefit from knowing what healthy options are available at the airports and restaurants they visit often. If you stay in a hotel regularly, see if you can get a room with a fridge, find a local grocery store and stock your room with healthy snacks and meals. It's just like keeping healthy food around at home; it just may take a little more effort.

On the flipside, if you're going on vacation, then you probably don't need to worry as much since it's a temporary departure from your usual routine. When you go back home, you'll return to your usual habits and the results will follow. The important ideas to remember when you're on vacation are: choose your indulgences wisely – have something special that you can't get at home, don't eat like crap just because "you're on vacation" – and make sure any less healthy choices you make while on vacation don't become habits when you're home. Get back on the horse.

FUEL BEFORE AND AFTER YOUR WORKOUTS

If you want to make the most of your workouts, you need to be eating and drinking. It's like putting gas in your car. Fueling before the workout will give your muscles the energy they need to work their best. Having something within 30 to 60 minutes after the workout will help your muscles recover faster, and maintain your strength-building, calorie-burning lean body mass. Since you're adding only one meal with this Habit, be sure that either your pre- or post-workout nourishment is a meal or snack that is already a part of your routine. For example, if you'll be exercising after work, you may need to add a small pre-workout snack at 4:00 PM, but can eat dinner as usual afterward at 7:30 PM. Here's a breakdown of what's best:

Before a Workout – Have a small snack and 16 oz. of water – that's the size of a regular Poland Spring bottle – one to two hours before exercising. The snack should be made of carbohydrates and a little protein. A few examples include a piece of fruit and low-fat string cheese, half a sandwich or a granola bar. If you work out first thing in the morning and are not very hungry, keep in mind that something is better than nothing. A small glass of juice or a piece of fruit should make a big difference. The key is to choose a snack that gives you energy, but does not make you feel like you're dragging a rock in your gut. If you feel heavy during your workout, next time eat your snack a little earlier or have a little less.

During a Workout – Drinking water is the key here. Aim for about four to six gulps of water every fifteen to twenty minutes while working out. Consider a sports drink only if your workout is greater than sixty minutes or if you're performing intense exercise in an extreme environment, such as very hot temperatures.

After a Workout – Fueling after your workout involves carbohydrates and protein again, although you may want a bit more food than you ate pre-workout. You're looking to get about a two-to-one ratio of carbs to protein. What does that mean? Half a turkey or peanut butter sandwich. Yogurt and a piece of fruit. A fruit smoothie made with a source of protein, like yogurt or milk. If you're short on time, go with a post-workout shake, such as a shaker bottle with whey protein, and a piece of fruit. A little something is always better than nothing. From a hydration standpoint, aim to drink about 16 to 24 ounces of fluid after your workout – that's a little more than one Poland Spring bottle. If those snack examples don't sound like the tastiest options, you can always craft your own snack using the information in the *What is a Balanced Meal or Snack* strategy on the next page.

ALWAYS HAVE SOMETHING HEALTHY HANDY

Think about the last time few times you were really hungry. Did you experience cravings or make less-than-ideal eating decisions? When you're famished, odds are you're more concerned with what you can eat immediately rather than what you can eat that's healthiest. To keep this from happening to you, stock healthy options everywhere your daily routine takes you. It's all about having food in places where you don't think you'll need it—until you do (and then you're grateful!):

- Keep a non-melting whole food or granola bar in your car.

- Carry a small bag of carrots, trail mix or a piece of fruit in your bag, briefcase or purse.

- Stock your desk at work with healthy snacks like nuts, whole grain cereal, peanut butter and fruit. And if you have a fridge at work, you can have things like low-fat string cheese, yogurt and hard boiled eggs too.

When you catch yourself starving somewhere, write down where and when it happened. Then plan how you can have a snack with you at that time in the future.

WHAT IS A "BALANCED" MEAL OR SNACK (AKA MINI-MEAL)?

Balanced Meals – If you're looking to do your body good with small, frequent meals, remember the slogan "Three every three." Based on a concept developed by Amanda Carlson-Phillips, VP of Nutrition and Research for Athletes' Performance and Core Performance, "three every three" means you should aim to eat the three main macronutrients - carbohydrates, fat and protein - every three to four hours.

Take a look at the Healthy Food Preference List in the Appendix for ideas on crafting a balanced meal based on healthy carbs or grains, lean proteins and fats. Choosing one from each section plus adding lots of fruit or veggies

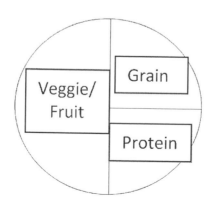

is a great way to create a healthy meal. When setting up your plate, focus on *mainly* plant-based whole foods (fruits and veggies, about 50% of the plate), a source of protein (which can include nuts, legumes, beans, etc., about 25% of the plate), whole grains or starchy veggies (about 25% of the plate) and healthy fats. Here are a few example meals with approximately that makeup:

BREAKFAST

- Oatmeal made with low-fat milk plus berries or raisins and almonds – cinnamon too
- Whole grain, low-sugar cereal with low-fat milk and a piece of fruit
- Scrambled egg sandwich on rye toast with avocado and tomato
- Smoothie with low-fat yogurt, fruit or veggies, avocado, ice and water

LUNCH

- Create-your-own sandwich with whole grain bread, lean protein such as turkey or chicken, and lots of veggies on top. Add in hummus or avocado as a sandwich topper, or a palmful of nuts on the side.
- Create-your-own salad with lots of different colored veggies, a lean protein such as tofu, grilled chicken or beans, and some avocado. Top with a little olive oil and vinegar or another low-calorie dressing.
- One slice of veggie pizza, a large side salad without cheese or croutons, low-calorie dressing and a piece of fruit

DINNER (QUICK RECIPES)

Chinese Beef with Broccoli

- 1/2 cup broccoli or broccoli slaw
- 1/4 cup onion and 1/4 cup carrot
- 3/4 cup snow peas
- 1/2 cup pineapple chunks
- 3 oz. lean beef (marinated, if desired)
- 1 tsp. sesame oil

- 2 Tbsp. low-sodium teriyaki sauce
- Garlic, ginger, crushed red pepper and black pepper to taste

Serve on 1 cup cooked brown rice

Tropical Salmon

- 4 oz grilled salmon
- 1 cup brown rice, cooked
- 1/2 cup black beans, drained
- Mango salsa with tomato, avocado, mango, lime, salt, pepper, jalapeno, etc.
- 2 cups veggies or greens sautéed with 2 tsp. olive oil and garlic

Fish Tacos

- 3 corn tortillas
- 3 oz. cooked fish
- Shredded lettuce or cabbage
- 1/4 avocado or 3 Tbsp. guacamole
- Tomato-based salsa and lime to taste

The Nightly Roast

- 4 oz. roasted beef or pork
- Baked potato with 2 Tbsp of low-fat sour cream
- 2 cups broccoli, asparagus or green beans cooked in 2 tsp of butter and tossed with a pinch of slivered almonds and lemon zest
- 1/2 cup fruit cocktail or applesauce

Crafting a Balanced Snack – A balanced snack is not a layer of chocolate, a layer of caramel and a layer of nuts. A balanced snack actually looks like a "mini-meal." The key is to choose a combination of foods that make you feel full, which is usually fiber, water, protein and/or healthy fats. The steps and food lists below can help you find food pairings that will keep you going strong between meals:

- *Step 1:* Choose a fruit, vegetable or grain. Choose fruits and veggies more often than grains.
- *Step 2:* Choose a lean protein or healthy fat.

Additional combinations:

- Fruit + Vegetable
- Vegetable + Grain + Fat (i.e. ½ veggie sandwich with hummus or avocado)

FOOD AND SNACK EXAMPLES

Fruits

- Handheld fruit like apples, bananas, pears, plums, nectarines, grapes
- Pre-cut fruit like pineapple, orange, melon, etc.
- Canned fruit in own juice (not syrup)
- Dried fruit (calories add up)

Vegetables

- Pre-cut veggies like celery, carrots, cucumber, red pepper spears, broccoli, etc.
- Veggies that can act as "wraps" like lettuce, cabbage, etc.

Grains

- Whole grain bread or crackers
- Rice cakes
- Popcorn
- Cereals low in added sugars (less than 5g per serving) & higher in fiber (> 3g per serving is best)

Lean Protein

- Low-fat string cheese
- Glass of low-fat or soy milk
- Yogurt
- Hardboiled eggs
- Low-sodium beef jerky
- Low-fat cottage cheese
- Leftover chicken/turkey

Healthy Fats

- Nuts/Seeds
- Hummus
- Nut butters
- Avocado

Some good combinations of these foods:

- Low-fat string cheese + apple
- Rice cakes with peanut butter
- Low-fat yogurt with a sprinkle of almonds or whole grain cereal
- Veggies with hummus
- Whole grain cereal with low-fat milk
- Low-sodium beef jerky and carrots
- Low-fat cottage cheese with fruit
- ½ sandwich (leftover poultry or peanut butter on whole grain bread or pita)

Pre- combined foods that make good snacks:

- Low-sodium, whole-food-based frozen meals, such as Amy's or Kashi
- Low-sodium soups
- Whole-food-based bars, such as Lara bar or Raw Revolution
- Lower-calorie granola bars, such as Kashi or Nature's Valley
- Trail mix

THE MEAL OF CHAMPIONS?

The debate over breakfast has been raging for years. Some say having breakfast daily, even a big one, can help with long-term weight loss; others say that a person will eat the same amount later in the day with or without the extra calories from a larger breakfast, which can result in weight gain. The jury is split. But instead of haggling over research, why don't we take a look at the people who've actually achieved the goal many of us are striving for: weight loss.

The National Weight Control Registry (NWCR) has been tracking the habits of over 10,000 people who have lost at least 30 pounds and kept it off for a year – people who've achieved significant, long-term weight loss. The NWCR has research findings that show 78% of those people eat breakfast daily. In other words, eating breakfast works for many, but not all. And they don't discuss what each person eats for breakfast. Much more research is needed in this area, actually.

My take on it is, treat breakfast like any other change in Habit #1: give it a shot for a few weeks and see how it impacts you the rest of the day, and ultimately how it impacts your results. If the thought of eating first thing in the morning is not very appealing, try building up your appetite gradually.

One thing that might help is that you don't need to eat the second you open your eyes. Take up to an hour to have your breakfast. Next, plan out what and how much you'll have – a meal with higher fiber and moderate protein may work best to keep you satisfied for the rest of the morning. Here are a few tips:

- For those who have no interest in eating in the morning but want to give breakfast a shot, start by drinking a big glass of water to get used to the feeling of putting something in your stomach (this helps with Habit #4 too!). Then you can move on to options with food.

- Want something quick, easy and not too heavy? This is where smoothies or meal replacement drinks can work in a pinch. Use fresh fruit or veggies for fiber, a source of protein and plenty of water or ice.

- Start small. Just like with anything else, your body doesn't like going from zero to 60 in the blink of an eye, so if you haven't been eating much for breakfast, start with something small like a piece of whole-grain toast and peanut butter, a small bowl of low-sugar cereal or a couple of scrambled eggs with veggies. Remember, fiber and protein.

- Make breakfasts that work for your lifestyle and get you the results that you want. Sustainability is key; actions become habits when you can perform them regularly, so go with the breakfast food choices that you can see yourself having on a regular basis and that leave you feeling satisfied and energetic.

KEEP EATING UNTIL TWO HOURS BEFORE BED

You can continue to eat until a couple hours before going to bed. You may have heard the "dieting rule" not to eat after a certain time, such as 7 PM. That one-size-fits-all statement is ridiculous, because it doesn't take into account whether you're going to bed at 9 PM or midnight! If you're going to bed at midnight, that's five hours between dinner and bed, and you should eat every three to four hours. So the 7 PM cut-off is only useful if you're in bed by 10 PM. You may be hungry around 10 PM if you last ate at 7, and in fact, you could have a small snack at that time if you're staying up till midnight. Just don't eat half a pizza. To calculate the last time you should eat each day, subtract two to three hours from your bedtime; that's about the right time to have your last mini-meal.

HABIT 2: EAT SMALLER MEALS

RATIONALE

The saying is absolutely true: Our eyes can be bigger than our stomachs. It was proven in a study by Brian Wansink, food marketing researcher at Cornell University and author of *Mindless Eating*: He had two groups of people – nutrition experts, actually! – enjoy an all-you-can-eat, no-time-limit ice cream social. There was only one difference between the two groups: One group was given smaller bowls and spoons to eat with compared to the other. Amazingly, the group with the larger bowls and spoons ate 30% more ice cream! That's a significant amount; it's 30% more calories they didn't need to eat.

So how much should you be eating at a meal? Unless you're trying to gain weight or you're an athlete under intense training conditions, you probably don't need more than 600-700 calories per sitting – even less, 300-500 calories, if you're a petite woman. Unfortunately, you can get at least 600 calories in one piece of restaurant cheesecake, a Five Guys'® cheeseburger or almost every Applebee's® appetizer as of June 2012. And let's not just pick on restaurants. Take a look around your own pantry and see how easily you can get up to 600 calories with your favorite dishes. One cup of cooked pasta or rice (the size of your fist) has about 200 calories. One ounce of cheese (the size of your thumb) has about 110 calories. The average bagel has about 300 calories…before any schmears or spreads. And any excess calories in your meal, whether they come from protein, carbs, fat or alcohol, go straight to body fat.

To make things worse, we often have to eat these meals faster than our bodies are designed to handle. Our high-demand work culture has led to lunch breaks of maybe 30 minutes which includes getting or preparing lunch, eating it, cleaning up and getting back to work. Then for dinner many of us get home so famished and exhausted from working late or shuttling kids around that the last thing on our minds is a well-balanced meal; we either get take-out or make something as fast as possible and shovel it in because we're starving.

The problem is that the body needs about 15 to 20 minutes to actually sense that it's full. That's why we'll eat like there's no tomorrow at the beginning of the meal, and then feel like we can't move a few minutes later. Our stomachs and brains finally caught up to our eyes and mouths. Do this enough times and the body won't even be able to pick up on the "hungry" or "full" signals anymore. Then it becomes easier and easier to eat more and more without realizing it. That's how people can eventually eat whole pizza pies and not get violently ill – they trained their body over time. Not a good type of training. Feeding your body when it's hungry (see Habit #1) and giving your body enough time to sense that it's full will help you manage your meal size.

ASSESSMENT

Track your eating habits using the Eating Habits Assessment form for three, four or seven days. The longer you track, the better. Include at least one weekend day, as eating habits are often different on the weekend. For this habit, focus on what time you ate, what foods you ate, portion size, hunger levels and energy levels , and how fast you ate or how much time you had to eat. Feel free to use things like your phone camera or Pinterest to track your eating habits with pictures; just be sure to label the information you need, such as energy and hunger levels, time, etc.

RECOMMENDATION

Aim to eat meals about 80% of the size of the meals from your assessment. That might mean serving yourself 20% less, or leaving about 20% of your meal on the plate. Then wait about 15 to 20 minutes for your body to detect satiety signals – that is, to catch up and see if it is still hungry. If you're really still hungry, then finish the rest of your meal or have a small snack. But if you feel satisfied, then you saved yourself a bunch of extra calories, and now have leftovers to eat the next day for lunch or dinner!

Or you can take an approach that the Okinawans in Japan have used for health and longevity: "Hara hachi bu," which means "eat until 80% full."

Either way, the goal is to make sure you're finishing meals satisfied, not stuffed. This loosely translates to finishing meals with a hunger level around 7 or 8 (on a 1 = starving to 10 = stuffed scale).

EASY EIGHT HABIT #2 STRATEGIES

SHRINK YOUR DINNERWARE

As Brian Wansink's ice cream socials demonstrated, our eyes can be bigger than our stomachs. But you can also make your mind believe you have more than enough food, even with smaller portions, by downsizing your plates, utensils and cups. For example, try eating your dinner from a salad plate, and cereal out of a coffee mug instead of a bowl, all with kids'-sized utensils.

Also, by putting less on your plate and using smaller utensils, it takes longer to eat the same amount of food, so your body has more time to sense that it's full. You don't want to finish each meal feeling that you can't possibly eat more; the meal is over when you simply don't feel hungry. And if you're compelled to clean your plate because of how you were raised, then smaller plates make it easier for you to fulfill that commitment without overeating.

LEAVE SOME FOOD ON THE PLATE – BUT NOT THE FRUITS OR VEGGIES

If you receive large portions away from home or aren't able to downsize your plates and bowls, leave some food on your plate at the end of the meal or have it packed up immediately for leftovers. If you're not used to doing this, just start with leaving a single fork or spoonful and slowly increase until about 10% to 20% of your meal is left. How much is that? Imagine your plate is like a pizza pie and cut it into eight slices. Try to leave about one slice's worth amount of food on the plate. Again, this is not forced deprivation, it's just another strategy to give your body the time it needs to feel if it's full. This also works for treats if you're prone to overindulging.

Wondering which foods to leave over? Not the fruits and veggies. They have the least calories, the most nutrients and usually fill you up the fastest due to their high water and fiber content. In fact, make it a point to eat your fruit, veggies or salad first, when you're most hungry and willing to eat them. Then move to the rest of the meal. If it's a combined meal like a stew or casserole, make sure all the veggies are gone from the plate when that 10% to 20% is left.

IF YOU'RE TRULY HUNGRY, HAVE A SNACK OR A LITTLE MORE FRUITS OR VEGGIES

In modern Western culture and workplaces, breaks and lunch times are limited or non-existent – so people eat as fast as they can or just skip the meal altogether. Emotional eating aside (to be addressed in Habit #5), most of the times you overeat come from eating too fast or from being starving after going too long without eating. Leaving 10% to 20% of your meal over is a built-in safety mechanism for those situations. If it's during the day and you're slammed with work or errands, leaving that bit of food over can prevent the sluggish mid-afternoon feeling of eating too much. And it gives you a snack to have later in the day so you're not starving before dinner.

If you find yourself starving at dinnertime, eat 80% of your meal and then see how you feel after 15 to 20 minutes. Call someone during that waiting time. Play with your kids. Do anything to get your mind off eating. The leftovers can be an evening snack if you're staying up late, or part of tomorrow's lunch.

TRY DRINKING BEFORE EATING (WATER, THAT IS)

Dehydration could also cause overeating. Your body is on a great quest for fluids, and it might signal you to eat excess food because a lot of foods contain water – but you also end up with those extra calories. Beyond that, since we're mainly made of water, dehydration is associated with decreased focus and increased stress to the body – that leaves you more susceptible to temptations and cravings. Fortunately, we have a zero-calorie solution for dehydration: water.

Drinking a glass of water before a meal serves two purposes. First, it rehydrates you so you can be sure you're eating because your body wants food, not fluid. Second, it will fill your stomach slightly so you'll feel full a bit faster. Getting full quicker will make it easier to leave over 10% to 20% of your meal, and you'll be less likely to overeat.

SHARE MEALS

Restaurant portion sizes these days can pack more than a day's worth of calories into just one meal, especially if you go for appetizers or dessert. If you really want a particular dish on the menu but don't want to eat all of it, get a little help from your friends. Asking someone to split a higher-calorie entrée or dessert with you lets you enjoy the food at half the calories.

OUT OF SIGHT, OUT OF MIND

A more subtle cause of overeating is picking at food after you're technically "done" with the meal. Sometimes it's because you're at an event where there's a continuous flow of food all night, such as a cocktail party or large potluck. Other times it happens while you're just sitting around the table. Imagine you're at a table talking with friends or family towards the end of dinner, and you've left over some pasta, fries or chicken on your plate. Then as you're chatting you glance at the food. Once you see it, you start thinking about eating again, even though you're not that hungry. So you have just one more piece, because it's there. And then another. Ten or fifteen minutes later you start wondering why you feel even more full than before, and that's when you look down at your plate. Clean.

Rather than having to resist picking at your food, nip your leftovers situation in the bud:

- Clear your dishes from the table as soon as you're done eating, and put leftovers in the fridge.

- Divide big batch meals into portions and put the extra away before serving, so you only have that night's portion available to eat. You can always get more if you're truly hungry.
- If you're at a restaurant, ask the server to take away your plate or bring you a to-go container as soon as you're done. If you know you'll be ordering a large meal, ask them to box half of the meal to go and serve the other half to you.
- Take deliberate steps to end your meal. Brush your teeth, chew gum, or drink a tall glass of water to cue yourself that the meal is over.
- If you're at a party, position yourself away from the food as soon as you're done eating.

HAVE ONE LESS COURSE

If you go out to eat often, how many courses do you typically eat? Do you always get an appetizer or a dessert? Or both? Do you often feel stuffed or bloated after going out to eat? Leaving 20% over does not always have to mean leaving food on the plate. It can mean just not having the plate at all.

Take stock of your current restaurant habits and then make a change. If you typically get an appetizer, entrée and dessert, drop one of them. If you just have an appetizer or a dessert, start splitting it with someone or just not having it at all – see how you feel with just an entrée. If you're still hungry, you could always order more food. Keep in mind that we're talking about your *habitual* restaurant meals, not occasional indulgences – unless indulgences are your habit. These tactics also work for home cooked multi-course dinners.

EAT SLOWER

Remember the adage, "Chew, chew, chew, chew, chew (and so on…) and swallow?" If you eat more slowly during a meal, you'll give your stomach the fifteen to twenty minutes it needs to sense it's full. A few other tips for eating more slowly during meal time:

- Put your fork, knife and/or spoon down between bites.
- Cut up your food into bite-sized pieces before you start eating. Re-

search shows that when you take more bites, you'll be satisfied with less food.

- Drink some water after every three bites.

- Make sure you're having a conversation during dinner. Talk about your day. Say more than, "It was good."

- Wait at least ten minutes between courses or before having seconds.

HABIT 3: EAT MORE FRUITS AND VEGGIES

RATIONALE

You can eat more and still lose weight. How is that possible? By focusing on *what* you're eating rather than *how much*. All you need to do is eat foods with higher nutrient density. The term *nutrient density* refers to how many nutrients a food provides compared to its calories. Nutrient density is essentially asking, "How many nutrients (fiber, vitamins, minerals, etc.) am I getting for the calories I'm consuming; what's the nutritional bang for my calorie buck?" Foods with more nutrients and fewer calories have a greater nutrient density. And what foods have the highest nutrient density? Fruits and veggies!

Here's a graph showing how all foods can be classified into one of four nutrient density categories:

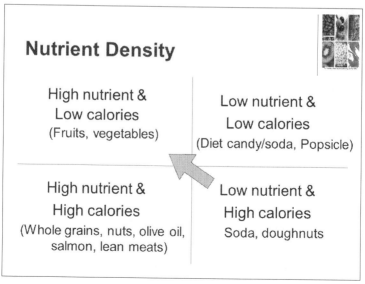

Nutrient Density

| High nutrient & Low calories (Fruits, vegetables) | Low nutrient & Low calories (Diet candy/soda, Popsicle) |
| High nutrient & High calories (Whole grains, nuts, olive oil, salmon, lean meats) | Low nutrient & High calories (Soda, doughnuts) |

To demonstrate the impact of nutrient density, I ask people at my nutrition seminars to compare their ability to eat meals of different nutrient densities. The first slide shows a quarter-pound fast food burger with cheese, medium fries and medium soda:

Nutrient Density

- Could you eat this at one sitting?

- Whopper with cheese
- Medium fries
- Medium soda

And then I ask, "Could you eat this meal at one sitting?" Most people, including myself, raise their hand. At some point in our lives we have all probably had a fast food meal. Then I show this slide:

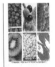

Nutrient Density

- How about this?

  - 2 Roasted Chicken Breasts w/ 2 Tbsp. BBQ Sauce
  - ½ lb. Lobster w/ ½ Tbsp Butter
  - 2 Sweet Potatoes w/ 1 Tbsp Brown Sugar and Cinnamon
  - 2 Cups Steamed Broccoli w/ Lemon
  - 2 Cups Spinach Sautéed in Garlic & 1 Tsp. Olive Oil
  - A 6" Turkey Subway Sub

And then I ask who could eat this meal at one sitting. Most people don't raise their hands for this one. And some people usually start saying "No way!" because they realize what the one similarity is between both meals...they are the same number of calories! About 1321 calories to be exact. This is how high calorie, low nutrient foods like burgers, fries and soda lead to weight gain. We can eat more of it and still not feel satisfied. On the other hand, the second list with more nutrient-dense foods can probably satisfy you for lunch, dinner and a snack or two.

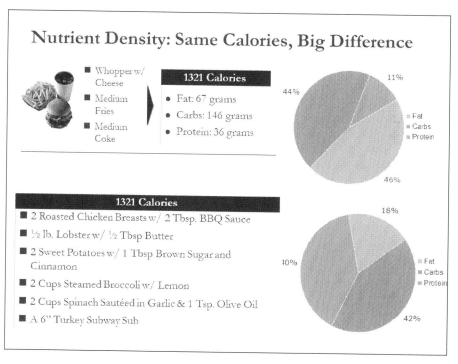

Nutrient Density: Same Calories, Big Difference

- Whopper w/ Cheese
- Medium Fries
- Medium Coke

1321 Calories
- Fat: 67 grams
- Carbs: 146 grams
- Protein: 36 grams

11%
44%
46%
Fat
Carbs
Protein

1321 Calories
- 2 Roasted Chicken Breasts w/ 2 Tbsp. BBQ Sauce
- ½ lb. Lobster w/ ½ Tbsp Butter
- 2 Sweet Potatoes w/ 1 Tbsp Brown Sugar and Cinnamon
- 2 Cups Steamed Broccoli w/ Lemon
- 2 Cups Spinach Sautéed in Garlic & 1 Tsp. Olive Oil
- A 6" Turkey Subway Sub

18%
10%
42%
Fat
Carbs
Protein

Here's another example. How many veggies you would have to eat to equal about 250 calories, the number of calories in an average candy bar:

- 1 cup of broccoli (31 calories)
- 1 cup of carrots (50 calories)
- 1 cup of celery (14 calories)
- 1 cup of cucumber (14 calories)
- 1 cup of cooked spinach (41 calories)

- 1 cup of cherry tomatoes (27 calories)
- AND about 2 or 3 tablespoons of Italian Dressing or Hummus to dip the veggies into! (80 calories or so)

*Calorie counts from CalorieKing.com

I'm not pointing this out to have you count calories or only eat vegetables for snacks. Instead I want to show *how much* food you can eat for the same number of calories. Heck, you could have half the candy bar and a cup of celery and still save 111 calories compared to eating the whole candy bar. Do that every day for a year and that's over eleven pounds of prevented weight gain.

We all know that we should eat less low nutrient, high calorie food. It turns out that adding in high-quality foods like fruits and veggies can be just as beneficial as eliminating unhealthy foods, though, because when we eat one thing, it usually replaces something else. For example, if you decide to have an extra serving of vegetables tonight at dinner, odds are you'll be full sooner, so you'll eat less of the pasta, rice, meat or soda that you're also having. Not only will you avoid eating all of those foods that have more calories than veggies, you'll be giving your body lots of added fiber, vitamins, minerals and water from the increased veggie intake.

For a more conscious substitution, you could have an apple, orange or pear with a yogurt or a palmful of nuts as your daily snack instead of a candy bar a few days a week. The change doesn't have to be at the same meal and same time every day, unless that works best for you (some of us like routines!). Having carrot sticks instead of chips at lunch one day and mixed berries instead of cookies as an after-dinner snack the next day is just as good as having the same healthy snack day after day. The key, of course, is to consistently eat that extra fruit or veggie at some point every day.

The most common reasons for not eating more fruits and veggies are that we don't like them, we don't know how to prepare them or we don't have ways to keep them fresh. But fear not, the answers are all here! This section is all about trying new fruits and vegetables as well as finding new ways to integrate them into your daily routine.

ASSESSMENT

Track which fruits and vegetables you eat, and how much of them, each day using the Fruit and Veggie Assessment Form for three, four or seven days. The longer you track, the better. Include at least one weekend day, as eating habits are often different on the weekend. For this habit, focus more on which and how much fruits and veggies you had (was it one slice of lettuce on a sandwich or a whole salad?), and when you had them. Feel free to use things like your phone camera or Pinterest to track your eating habits with pictures; just be sure to label the information you need, such as the time, associated meal or snack, fruit or veggie portion size, etc.

RECOMMENDATION

Starting with your baseline fruit and veggie intake, aim to eat two more servings of fruit and two more servings of veggies each week. That's four more servings of fruits and veggies per week.

Or if you're up for a challenge, aim to eat one more fruit or veggie each day. This would mean having seven more per week. Try doing half fruit, half vegetables to get the widest range of nutrients. For example, have an extra serving of veggies four days a week and an additional piece of fruit three days.

EASY EIGHT HABIT #3 STRATEGIES

READ THE HEALTHY FOOD PREFERENCE LIST

There's an extensive list of fruits and veggies in the Healthy Food Preference List in the Appendix. See which ones you like, dislike and have never tried. The ones you like are your go-to ideas for adding more fruits and veggies. You can also try one new fruit or veggie you've never had before each week, and see what you think of it. You may add a few more options to the rotation!

EAT THE RAINBOW

"Eat the Rainbow" is another great rule of thumb, courtesy of Amanda Carlson-Phillips at Athletes' Performance, for determining which fruits or veggies to eat each day or when making a salad or stir-fry. The color of each fruit or vegetable comes from the nutrients contained within it, so getting a range of colors gives you a range of nutrients that can promote everything from an improved immune system to lower cardiovascular disease risk. Here are a few examples for each color:

- **Green** – Green beans, cucumbers, snow peas, avocado, kiwi, honeydew melon
- **Red** – Red pepper, radishes, beets, cherries, red grapes, watermelon, strawberries
- **Yellow** – Yellow pepper, corn, yellow squash, lemons, golden apples, yellow pears
- **Orange** – Carrots, pumpkin, sweet potato, cantaloupe, peaches, tangerines
- **White/Tan** – Garlic, ginger, jicama, onions, potatoes, cauliflower, bananas
- **Blue/Purple** – Eggplant, assorted purple veggies (potatoes, peppers, etc.), blackberries, plums, blueberries
- *Many more listed in the Healthy Foods Preference List*

You can mix and match the different fruits and veggies to create meals and snacks with a range of nutrients in one tasty package:

	Rainbow Salad	Rainbow Stir Fry	Rainbow Fruit Salad
GREEN	Arugula	Broccoli	Avocado
RED	Red Pepper	Red Onion	Strawberries
YELLOW	Corn	Yellow Pepper	Pineapple
ORANGE	Carrots	Carrots	Mango
WHITE/TAN	Jicama or Onion	Garlic & Ginger	Banana
BLUE/ PURPLE	Blueberries or Olives	Eggplant	Blueberries

GREAT GREENS

What "superfood" does Popeye turn to when he needs to defend his fair maiden Olive Oyl? Spinach! Maybe it's because he knows that almost half of the calories in spinach come from protein. Or, he could go with kale: one cup provides more than 100% of your daily need for vitamins A, C and K along with a good dose of folate, B vitamins, copper, manganese and fiber—all wrapped up in a little 33-calorie package. Dark, leafy greens like spinach and kale also help prevent chronic diseases like cardiovascular disease and cancer.

The problem is that if I gave you a big bunch of greens and told you to eat up, would you take a bite? Or throw them back at me? Many people are at a loss for what to do with greens, especially the heartier ones, such as kale, collard greens and Swiss chard. Unless you can chow down on kale like a bunny (which is possible, I've done it…a little crunchy but slightly sweet), working these greens into your usual recipes and dishes is the best way to eat more of them. Here are some ways to get bunches of greens into your diet in a tasty, satisfying way:

Smoothies – If you're not a big fan of eating greens, try drinking them. When blended with fruit, ice and some milk or yogurt, even the most rugged greens become smooth and tasty – or tasteless, if you prefer. Regular blenders can do a good job with softer greens such as spinach, parsley, cilantro or watercress. A high-powered blender is better for tougher greens, such as kale and collard greens.

Omelets – Spinach is an especially good green to add to omelets. Other yummy options include arugula, beet greens and parsley. The key is to choose greens that soften quickly, but do not release too much liquid. There's a link to an omelet recipe in the Appendix with turnip greens, goat cheese and chili!

Grilled – Radicchio – not technically green, but still a very nutrient-dense leafy vegetable – and endive are great to throw on the grill after lightly brushing them with olive oil and sprinkling on some pepper. Serve with flavorful companions such as roasted peppers, olives and herbs.

Pasta sauce – Heartier greens, such as collards and kale, will cook down and soften while the sauce is simmering, giving it more texture. Chop the greens into bite-size pieces for the best results. Like pesto? You can make it chock full of greens, such as basil, parsley or even a little spinach—just go easy on the olive oil, pine nuts and cheese for a lower-fat version.

Baked – Baked kale chips are amazingly fast, easy and healthy! Simply wash the kale, tear it into bite-size pieces, and toss them with a little olive oil and a pinch of salt. If you want to spice it up you can even add some curry powder. Once the kale is evenly coated with the olive oil and spices, spread it across a baking sheet. Bake at 350° F for ten to fifteen minutes until the kale is crispy and enjoy! You also can bake kale into Italian classics like lasagna – that recipe is in the Appendix .

Soups and stews – Many classic soups and stews include dark, leafy greens such as kale, mustard greens and turnip greens. Like pasta sauces, soups and stews are cooked for a long time, so the greens can soften and provide a texture and taste to contrast the other ingredients. Greens go especially well in tomato-based stews, or soups with beans.

Sautéed – Whether sautéed with bacon or lentils, collard greens create the foundation of some classic side dishes. Try sautéing kale or Swiss chard with a little olive oil, fresh garlic, lemon zest and a dash of Romano or Parmesan cheese for a satisfying Italian-style side. The sweet, savory and spicy flavors from the pine nuts, raisins and red pepper flakes in Sautéed Greens with Pine Nuts and Raisins nicely complement the slightly bitter component of the greens – that recipe is in the Appendix.

Shredded – When shredded finely, even tougher greens become easy to handle. You can shred greens for a healthy garnish on mashed potatoes, or mix them into your favorite coleslaw recipe. Use a combination of shredded greens, like kale and parsley, with some quinoa, mint, lemon juice and olive oil to make a simple, tasty tabbouleh.

Wraps – Crunchy greens that contain a good amount of water, such as Swiss chard, bok choy, escarole or romaine lettuce, make fantastic wraps for a variety of fillings ranging from roasted eggplant with tomatoes, onion and garlic to teriyaki chicken with mandarin oranges.

Links to example recipes are listed in the Appendix.

**Note: If you are on anticoagulant therapy, such as Coumadin®, please speak with your physician before significantly changing your intake of dark, leafy greens.

MAKE FRUITS AND VEGGIES INTO SNACKS

During regular meal times, fruits and veggies can sometimes become lost in the mix and never get eaten. There's that bit of lettuce and tomato on top of a sandwich. Or the little side salad next to a big plate of meat and grains. Of course something's better than nothing, but why not let fruits and veggies have a starring role? That's where snacks come in.

Fruits and veggies are a good starting point for any snack. Check out the "Crafting a Balanced Snack" Tip for Habit #1, Eat More Often. You can pair fruits with peanut butter or yogurt. You can team up veggies with hummus, guacamole or a low-calorie dressing. Or you can just snack on them solo. The fiber and water content from produce, paired with a healthy fat or lean protein, can keep you full and satisfied, especially if you typically go six or more hours between meals – eating lunch at noon and dinner at 7:30 PM, for example.

MAKE FRUIT AND VEGGIES THE FIRST THING YOU EAT AT A MEAL

This is a great strategy for not only eating more fruits and veggies, but enjoying them more as well, especially if you come to a meal ravenously hungry. A question my colleague Adam Gilbert often asks his clients when they are trying to gauge their hunger level is: "Are you hungry enough, right now, to eat an apple?"

In other words, when you're truly hungry, the first thing you eat will be delicious, no matter what it is – so you might as well have that first thing be a fruit or veggie! When you belly up to the table for your meals, eat the fruits and veggies first. And then enjoy the rest of the meal.

Having the fruit and veggies first has two beneficial effects: it slows you down and makes you fuller faster. Fruits, veggies and salads take a while to chew, especially compared to foods like rice or pasta, which we can shovel into our mouths in seconds. So by taking the time to chew, chew, chew on your produce, you get closer to the fifteen to twenty minutes needed for your body to realize it's actually full. Finally, fruits and veggies have lots of water, fiber and nutrients that can make you feel full during a meal faster than other foods.

A LAUNDRY LIST OF WAYS TO GET MORE FRUITS AND VEGGIES

Intending to eat more fruits and veggies is one thing, but a lot of people draw a blank on exactly how to do it. A produce "writer's block," if you will. Fear not, below are a bunch of ways you can add fruits and veggies to your meals throughout the day:

Breakfast

- Grab a piece of fruit in the morning, along with your whole grain roll or English muffin and coffee or tea.
- Add two handfuls of berries to your morning cereal.
- Add chopped vegetables, such as tomato, mushrooms, onion, spinach or peppers, to your scrambled eggs or breakfast sandwich.
- Add fresh fruit, such as banana or berries, to your pancake or French toast recipe. Top with sliced apples.
- Make your own fresh-fruit smoothie with some skim milk or yogurt and ice. Add some vegetables to the mix, such as cucumber, cilantro, or tomato, for extra nutrients with a mild flavor.
- If you drink juice, choose 100% juice without added sugars or fillers. And keep the serving size down to a small glassful.
- Add almonds, berries or apple chunks and cinnamon to your oatmeal.

Lunch

- Top your sandwich with lots of fresh vegetables, such as romaine lettuce or spinach, tomato, onions, sprouts, mushrooms or fresh red pepper. They add flavor and a nice crunch.
- Choose a soup loaded with vegetables, such as minestrone, chicken

with vegetables, or carrot ginger.

- Bring along a handful of baby carrots, celery spears, or a piece of fruit to munch on with your lunch.

- Add fruit to your salads, such as apples, pears, or oranges, for a sweet and tangy kick.

- Get veggies, fruit or a salad as your side dish rather than chips or fries.

Dinner

- Add some chopped vegetables, such as carrots, mushrooms, or peppers, to your mashed potatoes. You'll barely notice them. Or try making mashed cauliflower – same flavor, less calories.

- Buy a bag of spinach and throw a handful on top of your dinner as a colorful garnish. The heat of your food will wilt the spinach, so it blends in and becomes a healthy addition with little extra effort.

- Roast vegetables while you cook everything else. Slice some vegetables, such as eggplant, peppers, onions and sweet potatoes, rub them with a little olive oil and spices and place them on a baking sheet. Bake at 400° F for 30-40 minutes, depending on thickness, while you cook the rest of your meal.

- The 7-minute sweet potato: Use a fork to poke a bunch of holes in a sweet potato. Place it in the microwave on high for 6-7 minutes, flipping the potato over once halfway through cooking. Cook it until you can easily slip a fork into it. Cut it open and top it with some cinnamon and low-fat yogurt. Use caution when you open it—these potatoes can get hot!

- If you're in the mood for pizza, buy one slice loaded with vegetables, instead of two plain slices. Add a side salad.

- If you're in the mood for Chinese, choose an option that has "mixed vegetables" or "broccoli" in the name. If you want to go one step further, get your dish steamed with sauce on the side.

- If you're in the mood for Mexican, add beans, peppers, onions and any other extra vegetables available, such as tomato, cilantro or fresh salsa.

IN SIGHT, IN MIND: KEEP 'EM AROUND

The best way to ensure you eat fruits and vegetables is to have them available around you:

- Always keep some stocked in the fridge at home or work. Baby carrots, grape or cherry tomatoes and many types of fruit are ready-to-eat. If you like big fruits like pineapple or melons, or vegetables like broccoli, celery or cucumber, cut it up into chunks or pieces as soon as you get home from the grocery store. You could even put them into individual plastic baggies so you can grab and go when you need a snack in a pinch.

- For those with little time, just add a fork or hand. You can always buy pre-cut fruits and vegetables such as celery pieces, broccoli florets, mixed fruit salads, etc. The produce aisle in supermarkets also has many other ready-to-go veggie and dip combo options – just make sure the dip isn't a calorie bomb.

- Get rid of the candy bowl at home and work. Instead keep a fruit basket stocked with oranges, apples, pears, bananas and even kiwis – cut kiwis in half and then eat the inside with a spoon.

- If all else fails, consider the can. The one thing that canned fruit has going for it is that it can sit around for a while and still be good, while fresh fruit goes downhill after a few days. But this increased shelf life comes at a price: canned fruit loses a fair amount of its nutrients during the packaging process…but it's still better than nothing. Make sure you buy fruit canned in its own juices, not in syrup. A can of fruit still has more nutrients and significantly fewer calories than a candy bar.

EAT THE FRUIT, DON'T DRINK THE JUICE

Ever wonder what the nutritional difference is between drinking 12 ounces of juice – a coffee-mug's worth – vs. eating the fruit itself?

Juice (12 oz.)	Calories	Fiber	Fruit (Medium)	Calories	Fiber
Orange	163	0	Orange	62	3.1
Apple	178	0	Apple	95	4.4
Pineapple	192	0	Pineapple (1 cup)	83	2.3
Grapefruit	150	0	Grapefruit	82	3
Grape	255	0	Grapes	104	1.5

A typical, 12-ounce serving of juice has about twice the number of calories as the fruit itself. And the juice has no fiber, while the fruit has at least a few grams per piece. Just switching from juice to whole fruit can save you eight to ten pounds per year. Small change, big impact.

HABIT 4: DRINK MORE LOW OR NO-CALORIE BEVERAGES

RATIONALE

To make health, fitness and weight improvements, don't just look at what you eat – think about what you drink. Beverages often have more calories than we realize. A pint of beer or a gin and tonic can have 175 calories or more, and it'll also send your body signals to hold onto fat around your waist. One can of soda has about 120 calories and zero nutrients. In fact, drinking just one less can of soda per day can save you up to ten pounds per year.

While soda and alcohol are obvious culprits, even supposedly "healthy" drinks like iced tea, lemonade and juice can pile on the calories quick. Most packaged iced teas, lemonades and fruit drink mixes have just as much sugar as soda. And eight ounces of most juices are about 100 calories. While juice does have more nutrients than the other beverages, the juicing process gets rid of most of the fruit's natural fiber. As a result, you need to drink more juice – and more calories – to feel satisfied. You can get more nutrients for fewer calories by eating the actual fruit!

Then there are the low-calorie beverages, like tea and coffee, that we turn into high-calorie bombs by adding lots of sugar and cream. Finally, unless you're training very hard or for more than sixty minutes at a time, you do not need the electrolytes or calories from sports drinks or nutrient- (and calorie-) enhanced waters.

On the other hand, staying hydrated throughout the day is essential for maintaining your energy and focus. About 60% of your body is made of water, and even a 1% decrease in hydration can have a negative impact on how you feel and function. Have you ever had a headache, were sluggish or felt hungry, and then felt your head clear after a drink of water? Staying hydrated minimizes stress on your body and helps you function better in all aspects of life: work, family, eating and physical activity.

Being dehydrated could also lead to eating extra calories you don't need, and then weight gain. Sometimes we will eat food when we are, in fact, thirsty rather than hungry. Your body is looking for that fluid one way or the other. So drinking some zero-calorie water would have given you the same satisfaction as eating a high-calorie snack. And if that snack is dry or salty, odds are you will become even thirstier and more dehydrated—a vicious cycle. The best thing to do is to have a drink and see if your hunger was a desire for food or fluid.

A rule of thumb for getting in enough fluids is to aim for half of your body-weight in ounces of fluids per day, with water being the best choice. For example, if you're 150 pounds, your target should be 75 ounces of fluid per day. That's about equal to four and a half regular 16-ounce Poland Spring bottles, or two and a quarter liters. You need more fluid than that if you're physically active, particularly before, during and after exercise.

ASSESSMENT

Track what types of fluid you drink each day, and how many ounces, using the Beverage Assessment Form. Track *everything* you drink for three, four or seven days. The longer you track, the better. Include at least one weekend day, as eating habits are often different on the weekend. Focus on when you drank the beverage, what beverage you consumed, how big it was (a 16-ounce water bottle, a 1 liter water bottle, a 20-ounce soda, etc.), any items you added like sugar or cream, and the beverage's "grade" as defined on the assessment form. Feel free to use things like your phone camera or Pinterest to track your eating habits with pictures; just be sure to label the information you need, such as time, added ingredients and "grade."

RECOMMENDATION

From your baseline beverage intake, improve your fluid intake by having one more low-calorie beverage each day, or by replacing one high-calorie beverage with a lower-calorie option each day – for example, replace a soda with a water, seltzer or unsweetened iced tea. If you have several high-calorie beverages each day, you can either rotate which you replace or choose to replace the same one every day.

EASY EIGHT HABIT #4 STRATEGIES

HYDRATE DURING YOUR WORKOUT

You need about half your body weight in ounces of fluids per day, and being physically active increases that demand. An easy way to make sure you get enough is to drink water before, during and after the workout so you don't have to make it up later on. Here are the basic recommendations:

- Drink 16 ounces of water one to two hours before exercising.
- Drink four to six ounces of water every fifteen minutes during exercise. That's about four to six gulps.
- Drink 16 to 24 ounces of water after exercise. Technically, you're supposed to have 16 ounces of water for every pound of weight lost during exercise, for those that are counting.

As a reminder, you should only have a sports drink like Gatorade or Powerade if you're planning on working out for more than 60 minutes, if your exercise routine is particularly intense or you're exercising in an extreme environment, like outside on a very hot day. Otherwise, cold water will do the trick.

WATER BOTTLE, MEET BAG

Camels carry water around with them all the time in their humps. Be like a camel. Carrying a water bottle with you wherever you go ensures you can stay hydrated anytime, anywhere. I recommend going with about a one-liter sized bottle, which is 32 ounces: big enough so you only have to refill it a couple times a day, but small enough so it doesn't feel like a ton of water weight (pun intended).

If lugging a big water bottle around is not your idea of fun, you could keep one at each of your usual locations instead: one at home, one at work, one in your car, etc. Then get a smaller one that you can keep in your bag or purse for when you're on the go. You could also buy a smaller water bottle for yourself at work so you have to get up more often throughout the day to refill it – less sitting time!

YOU CAN MAKE WATER TASTE BETTER

Water doesn't have to be tepid, lukewarm and bland. Let's hear that one again: water does not have to be a forced, unpleasant drink…if you choose to make it appealing. Here are some tips:

- *Make it cold* – You can keep it in the fridge, add ice cubes or even freeze it overnight and then drink the melting, cold water throughout the day.

- *Add a splash of flavor* – Add some lemon or lime to your ice-cold water – you can squeeze it fresh yourself, or use those little squeeze-bottles. Or you can soak some other fruits, veggies or spices in water overnight for a unique taste. Try chopped berries, cucumber slices, wedges of citrus fruit or sage. Chill it in the fridge overnight and enjoy the next day! If you usually drink juice, try doing 50/50 water and juice, or just add a splash of juice, to get more water in. I also recently came across a useful product called True Lemon; packets of crystallized lemon that add flavor without any artificial sweeteners. They make other citrus flavors as well.

- *Make it fizzy* – If you like carbonated drinks, try sparkling water or seltzer. Feel free to make it cold and add flavors. Or you can make your own with appliances like the Sodastream. Seltzer has the same number of calories as water: zero.

- *Have water with meals and snacks* – Many people want to taste something when they drink a beverage. That's why you may prefer adding lemon or lime, or drinking things other than water. So rather than having water on its own, drink it with meals or snacks to get the flavor of food between gulps. Having water with meals is helpful in two ways: it fills your stomach up so you may eat less, and taking consistent sips of water should slow down your eating. Remember, it takes fifteen to twenty minutes for your body to register that it's full.

If you have 16 ounces of water – about the size of a regular Poland Spring bottle – with every meal and snack, then you'll drink 48 to 96 ounces of water a day depending on how many meals you have. You can save your flavored beverages for between meals when you'll likely enjoy them more.

DRINK ACCORDING TO PLAN, OR AT LEAST WHEN YOU'RE THIRSTY

Try creating a hydration plan. Once you've done the Beverage Assessment and gotten a good idea of your baseline habits, see where you can easily add in another glass or two of water during the day. Here are a few ideas:

- Have a glass of water when you wake up.
- Have a glass of water with each meal or snack.
- Have a drink of water or other low-calorie beverage every thirty to sixty minutes at work.
- Have a glass of water or low-calorie beverage before bed at night.
- Create an automated reminder in your phone or planner to have a glass of water.

If this seems like too much work, just make it a point to have a glass of water every time you feel thirsty. Thirst is an indicator that you're getting dehydrated, so listen to your body. Otherwise your body will let you know quite quickly: less energy, trouble focusing, headache and increased craving for food. Who knew that fluids can cure so many ills?

EAT YOUR CALORIES, DON'T DRINK THEM

These days it's very easy to consume extra, needless calories via beverages. At least eating calories requires chewing! Here are some facts about how higher-calorie beverages can lead to unwanted pounds:

Soda – The average soda bottle is now twenty ounces, contains about 250 calories and has zero natural nutrients. I'm sure some company will eventually add vitamins and minerals to soda and call it "healthy soda," just like the sugary, nutrient-enhanced waters currently on the market. Soda has no redeeming qualities. It's useless. If you drink soda regularly, reducing the amount you drink by one can or bottle a day would be an excellent habit change. If you drink one bottle a day, see if you can cut back to half a bottle and pour out the rest. If you feel uneasy about "wasting" soda, save it for the next day, buy a smaller portion – one of those mini eight-ounce cans – or save yourself $1 to $1.50 by skipping the soda entirely!

If you like the fizz of soda but don't want the calories, have some flavored seltzer or sparkling water. If you really need something sweet, you can substitute a sports or nutrient-enhanced drink like Gatorade or Vitamin Water – these aren't particularly healthy, but they do typically have half the number of calories per serving than soda. This substitution can eventually lead to drinking water if you use half sports drink/half water and eventually transition down to just water. If soda is a must, have less of it or try alternating between a glass of soda and a glass of water to reduce your total sugar and calorie intake.

Sports Drinks/Nutrient-Enhanced Waters – These beverages typically have 125 calories per twenty ounce bottle, and are only designed for people who are being very physically active. The isolated vitamins that are added to these drinks are fairly useless unless they're consumed with actual food. And if you want to supplement your daily meals with extra nutrients, just take a multivitamin for 125 fewer calories and probably 90% less cost.

Energy drinks – Similar calories (a lot) and nutrient (none) profile to soda, plus added stimulants and maybe a few added, isolated vitamins. And by the way, some of these stimulants may be regulated by athletic commissions like the International Olympic Committee. If some of the fittest people shouldn't be having these substances, why should you?

If you need these drinks to keep you alert, go with a cup of coffee. Or a good night's sleep. If you like the flavor or fizziness, try downgrading the calorie intake with either seltzer plus a splash of juice or a sports drink (has fewer calories and sugar than energy drinks). You can also reduce your intake of energy drinks using the same methods as you would for soda.

Juice – While juice has some nutrients, it comes with a lot more calories and less fiber than the fruit itself. Check out the section *Eat the Fruit, Don't Drink the Juice* in Habit #3 for more details. If you're going to have juice, keep the portion small, or simply try eating the fruit itself. You could also do a "light" version of the juice by using half the amount of juice you normally use and adding the other half as water. You could do 75% juice and 25% water to start if you find it's too bland.

Coffee – One or two daily cups of coffee the size of a regular coffee mug is fine. A single Grande coffee from Starbucks is the equivalent of two regular-sized cups. When you start downing more than two cups of coffee a day, the caffeine can impact everything from your heart to your brain and even your sleeping habits—even if you don't actually feel a caffeine buzz. If you find yourself living on coffee all day, try cutting back one cup at a time to avoid withdrawal symptoms. Anyone who suddenly quits drinking large amounts of coffee cold turkey can confirm that caffeine is addictive at higher levels...so it's better to wean yourself off gradually.

Now let's talk about the coffee culprits: the sugar and milk. At my local coffee shop I've counted as people pour sugar into their cups of coffee for upwards of eight to ten seconds! As a former engineering nut, I decided to measure how much sugar ended up in those drinks: I poured sugar onto a napkin for eight seconds. About one packet of sugar, or one teaspoon, came out of the shaker per second, which means eight to ten packets were added in as many seconds.

Each sugar packet is about 15 calories, so those people were adding 120 to 150 calories from pure sugar! If they then poured in milk, half- and-half, or cream, they added another 50-100 calories or more. So our daily cup of coffee becomes a 200-calorie drink! No need to change overnight, but if you currently use six packets of sugar and a load of cream in your coffee, this is a good place to start making changes…one packet at a time.

Finally, don't even get me started on mocha/frappe/latte drinks. Seems like the more words in the name of the drink, the more calories that are in it. While a basic low-fat latte has about 140 calories, some of those sweetened, creamy drinks have as many calories as a meal: 400 to 600 calories for the large sizes!

If you buy any drinks loaded with milk or sugar, try downgrading. Use low-fat milk instead of whole. Have a smaller size. Ask for fewer pumps of syrup or add fewer sugar packets. Low-fat or non-fat cappuccinos and lattes have the least calories of the coffee drinks, though they still usually have about 80 to 140 without any added sugar. Black coffee or a shot of espresso have about five calories, and each packet of sugar has about 15 more, so you can have coffee with two packets of sugar and a splash of low-fat milk for about 50-60 calories.

Alcohol – The average drink, which is twelve ounces of beer, five ounces of wine or 1.5 ounces of liquor, is equal to about 90 to 140 calories. And don't forget about the mixers! Some higher-calorie mixers like soda, juice and tonic can add another couple hundred calories. Believe it or not, tonic water has similar amounts of sugar to soda – it just doesn't taste as sweet because of the bitter quinine. Commercial or restaurant frozen mixed drinks like daiquiris, margaritas and mudslides are the worst of all – the added sugar, fat and alcohol can set you back as many calories as an entire meal: 400 calories or more. If you want a better frozen drink, replace mixes with the real thing. For example, instead of strawberry daiquiri mix and ice, use real frozen strawberries.

Not only does alcohol have lots of calories, it also causes your body to hold onto fat. Your body views alcohol as a toxin, so it focuses on burning the alcohol instead of whatever you just ate or are about to eat. As a result, all of that food is stored on you rather than burned. And because alcohol increases stress hormones such as cortisol, those calories are more likely to be stored as fat…

around your belly. Finally, don't forget about the extra calories from any poor food choices made while buzzed – all food looks good when you've been drinking.

If you do choose to drink, aim for one drink at a sitting for women and no more than two for men – one drink equals one beer bottle, five ounces of wine (about one-fifth of a regular bottle) or a shot glass of liquor (1.5 ounces). A great trick is to alternate one drink with a glass of water, which will help prevent dehydration, make you fuller sooner and hopefully allow the night to pass with minimal alcoholic drink consumption. Avoid high-calorie mixers like frozen drinks, soda, juice and tonic. Instead order dark beer (you'll drink it slower), a glass of red wine, or a drink "on the rocks," with a twist or with a water or seltzer mixer. Set a drink limit before you go out and stick to it. Cut yourself off or get a stiff drink for your last one so you can "nurse" it the rest of the night. If you feel pressured to continue drinking when you'd rather stop, go "stealthy healthy" by ordering a seltzer with a twist of lime. Looks like a drink, but isn't.

It's worth putting in the effort to drink less alcohol – one less drink per week will save you at least two pounds per year. Five less drinks…ten pounds.

WHAT ABOUT "DIET" DRINKS?

This is the classic double-edged sword. Many people who crave something sweet or fizzy with food turn to diet soda or other diet drinks. I did too for a long time; in high school and college I had three or four diet sodas per day. However, research has been coming out showing that diet soda may not actually suppress our sweet tooth…in fact, it may make you crave even more sweet foods or drinks, and lead to weight gain instead of the weight loss most dieters are going for! Here are two theories about the ineffective sweetness of diet beverages:

1. Our body has been primed to receive something sweet, but it didn't get the calories associated with the sweetness since diet soda has zero calories. So it now wants to satisfy this newly created calorie craving by eating something else, or eating more.

2. These extremely sweet artificial sweeteners blunt our body's ability to detect and become satisfied from the natural sugars found in fruit, dairy, etc. Therefore we need to add more and more sugar – and calories – to our foods to become satisfied. Feeling is believing: get a piece of fruit and a diet beverage. Eat half the fruit and note how sweet it is. Then drink the diet beverage and have the other half of the fruit. Sense how the sweetness changes.

Also, diet sodas are made with artificial sweeteners that have been linked to cancer. While the government considers the level of these chemicals in diet soda as safe for human consumption, I don't think it's worth the risk if you're willing to choose a different option. While sugar isn't ideal, at least it's a known hazard. There's also been a big push to use the Stevia plant as a low-calorie natural sweetener. My jury is still out on Stevia. In the end, it's best to wean yourself off the need for these "sugar highs" as much as possible. Aiming to have less intense sweetness, whether natural or artificial, is the best goal. The key is to make all changes gradual and consistent.

Am I going to say you should never have a diet soda, diet iced tea or other diet beverage? No, because then I'd be a hypocrite. I'm down to about two or three cans of diet soda per week. I drink diet soda now and then because I like the taste and don't want the calories. Other people would rather avoid the artificial sweeteners, which is fine as long as you can burn off the calories.

These are my thoughts on diet drinks, both as a dietitian and as a person:

- If you don't drink diet sodas or other diet beverages now, there's no need to start.
- If you do drink diet beverages, have them in moderation – a few times a week or once a day at most, not five per day. If you feel that you're having too many, reduce gradually. Have one less for a couple of weeks until you get used to it. Then reduce it again by one for another few weeks and so on until you get to a moderate number.
- If you currently drink regular soda or other high-calorie beverages, and you don't want to switch directly to water or another low-calorie

drink, diet drinks could be a step along the way – as long as you have them in moderation, one per day or less. If this is you, the diet drinks should be a direct swap for the higher-calorie option. But make sure you don't compensate by eating more.

- If you're diabetic, you're more susceptible to the impacts of large hits of sugar from drinks like regular soda, iced tea and fruit drinks, so diet beverages might be your go-to drink. Yet artificial sweeteners can have similar consequences for diabetics – it can overstimulate your body's sweetness receptors and cause you to overeat afterwards. Like everyone else, see if you can have less diet soda and more water.

BEYOND WATER: OTHER LOW-CALORIE HYDRATION OPTIONS

Besides water, your best drink options have few or zero calories, no artificial sweeteners and ideally give you some nutrients for the calories you're drinking:

Sparkling water or seltzer – A great option if you like the fizzy feeling of soda. You can find plenty of naturally-flavored options, or you can flavor it yourself with things like lemon juice. Beware of artificially sweetened sparkling waters that have the same issues as diet soda.

Unsweetened tea, green tea or iced tea – Use lemon juice or a little bit of sugar to make it more palatable. Since one packet of sugar has about fifteen calories, and typical commercial iced tea mixes and bottles have six to eight times that amount, you're better off adding your own packet or two of sugar. The same goes for commercial lemonade and fruit-flavored drinks. In the long run, no sugar is best, but better to control the amount yourself! Keep in mind that green and black teas have caffeine, though not as much as coffee. If you want to avoid caffeine, go with herbal teas.

Coffee – In moderation, one or two small cups of coffee are fine and may even have some benefits. Just be sure to limit how much milk and sugar you add and try to drink your coffee in the morning, because caffeine later in the day could cause poor sleep quality that night.

Low-fat dairy and smoothies – While these drinks have calories, they also provide you with nutrients such as calcium and protein, and fiber from any fruit you add, which keep you fuller longer than other beverages. Drink these as part of a snack, as a meal replacement or for post-workout refueling.

HABIT 5: INDULGE LESS FREQUENTLY

RATIONALE

The Habit #3 approach of having more of the good stuff – fruits and veggies – is one way to eat more healthily, but some people may prefer to focus on eating less of the not-so-good stuff instead. This means adjusting how often they indulge in foods with low nutrient density. These foods provide very few nutrients in a high-calorie package. Some common examples include fried foods, pastries, ice cream, alcohol and triple bacon cheeseburgers. Here are the four questions to ask yourself when dealing with indulgences:

Question One: "What am I indulging on?" – Sometimes we're unaware of how many high-calorie foods we're eating, because we don't consider them to be "junk food." But a lot of foods with fairly good reputations are actually low-nutrient-density indulgences. For example, did you know that a cup of granola has about 500-600 calories while a cup of most other cereals have 150-200 calories? Or that the average bagel has about the same number of calories as three to four slices of bread? You could save about a hundred calories a day by using two slices of bread for your morning sandwich instead of a bagel.

Question Two: "How often am I indulging?" – Sometimes I ask my clients how often they indulge, and they tell me, "Not very much at all. I only have pizza one night a week. And I only have a burger and fries one day a week. I only get a doughnut for breakfast once per week; otherwise I just have a bagel with cream cheese. On the weekends I'm a little less strict because we go out to eat more and I only drink on the weekends, about three beers each evening. And then I..."

A few smaller indulgences throughout the week or one indulgent meal on the weekend does not ruin a healthy lifestyle. Frequent indulgences can have a negative impact, however, because frequent indulgences become indulgent habits. And our habits become our results.

By the way, that client's bagel with cream cheese usually has more calories than his doughnut!

Question Three: "How much am I having when I indulge?" – When you indulge, is it a meal like a burger and fries? Or a side like some macaroni and cheese? Or a slice of cake at the end of a healthy, balanced dinner on Saturday night?

Or is it half a pizza? Or a pint of ice cream? Or a multi-course extravaganza with appetizer, entrée, dessert and half a bottle of wine?

Again, one big indulgence does not completely derail progress, especially if we're able to get back on the right track as soon as we become aware that we've indulged heavily. However, the bigger the indulgence, the less frequently it needs to occur to have a negative impact. For example, you may be better off having a couple small cookies every night after dinner (150 calories x 7 days = 1050 calories per week) rather than having a huge buffet, a multi-course feast or going on a drinking binge every Saturday night (2000+ calories per week).

Question Four: "Why am I indulging?" – We choose to indulge for lots of reasons: comfort, family, friends, happiness, lifestyle or stress. Many times people indulge because it provides them with pleasure: it could be a special occasion such as a birthday, vacation or wedding. Other times it's just built into their routine, such as going out for drinks and dinner every Saturday night with friends. You may consider yourself a "foodie," for example, where cooking and enjoying indulgent food is a part of your lifestyle.

Whatever the reason, food plays an important role in your life and that's not to be taken lightly. However, ask yourself whether the foods you enjoy also prevent you from enjoying other aspects of life, such as feeling energetic, being active, staying healthy or looking trim. The goal is to create a balance that gives you the best overall quality of life: food, fitness and feelings.

Last but certainly not least, sometimes people eat when they don't really need to or want to as a way to cope with emotions, guilt or stress. Emotional eating is a significant issue that will be addressed in this Easy Eight Habit strategies section.

ASSESSMENT

Track your indulgences using the Indulgence Frequency Assessment forms for three, four or seven days. The longer you track, the better. Include at least one weekend day, as eating habits are often different on the weekend. For this habit, focus on when you indulged, what food you indulged in, how much of it you had, the reason for indulging, the level of satisfaction you felt from the indulgence and the intensity of the indulgence. The form has an "indulgence scale" to help you assess and compare the intensity of your indulgences. The scale is based on the nutrient density of the food and the quantity consumed.

RECOMMENDATION

Based on your Indulgence Frequency Assessment and Indulgence Details Tracker, decrease your indulgences by either one intense indulgence or two less-intense indulgent foods per week. Sometimes it's just a matter of making big indulgences smaller, such as having a scoop of ice cream instead of a pint, or having two slices of pizza instead of half a pie.

Substitution, omission, preparation and distraction are four ways you can replace an indulgence. You'll find tips for each of those below, along with other strategies for dealing with cravings, temptations and emotional eating.

EASY EIGHT HABIT #5 STRATEGIES

CREATE INDULGENCE ALTERNATIVES

Sometimes we indulge because we want to, but other times we indulge because "it just happened to be there." Take responsibility for both your actions and your environments, so you can indulge on your own terms. Otherwise you'll be more vulnerable to changes in your environment beyond your control, such as when someone brings in a big batch of cookies from home and you aren't prepared with your healthy mid-afternoon snack at work. Other times, you already know that certain circumstances or environments create indulgent responses no matter what you do. For example, you may know that no pint of Ben & Jerry's will last more than two days in your home.

Read through your assessment to get a feel for the circumstances surrounding your temptations, and figure out what adjustments will allow you to indulge on your own terms. Here are four methods you can use to change your future responses to an indulgence or temptation:

1. *Omission – Get temptations or cravings out of sight, and therefore out of mind.*

- Make sure tempting foods are not around you. If you know that the smell or sight of a chocolate chip cookie turns you into a human Cookie Monster, make your house, desk at work or any other place you spend time a "no cookie zone." This way you can truly enjoy the cookie you have every now and then at a café or restaurant, rather than feel guilty about cookies you eat every day.

- Ask your co-workers or friends not to include you when they're ordering from fast-food restaurants, and make it a point to go only to restaurants with healthier options when you go out to eat.

2. *Substitution – Making a healthier choice, or having a healthier choice available, in response to a temptation or craving.*

- Do you always need something sweet after dinner? Rather than a high-calorie piece of cake or cookies, try a piece of dark chocolate or a date stuffed with an almond or pecan (tastes like pecan pie!). Or if you need something cold and sweet, try a frozen fruit bar or low-fat frozen yogurt instead of ice cream. In the end, these options will only stick if they satisfy you. Otherwise just have less of your preferred indulgent foods.

- A stressful day at work? Rather than coping with your day via a pastry, think up some alternatives: Problem-solve your work issues, go to a yoga class, meditate or just sit up tall and focus on taking ten deep breaths slowly through your stomach.

3. *Preparation – If you know that you're going to have to deal with temp-*

tations or cravings, plan ahead to give yourself options to make a better choice.

- Starving from going six hours between meals? Bring a satisfying snack with you from home, such as carrots and hummus, or yogurt and a few almonds, so you can turn down the free junk food being offered at work at 3 PM. Or if your commute is long, you can have it on the way home to keep you from gorging at dinner.

- If you know you're going out to a less healthy restaurant or fast food establishment, read the menu ahead of time and find the healthiest dishes that will satisfy you. This will keep you focused and resistant to temptation when you get there and smell that triple cheeseburger or see that creamy pasta option on the menu.

4. *Distraction – Do something that will get your mind off of the temptation or craving.*

- Bored at work and getting hungry? Try drinking water – maybe you're actually thirsty – or getting up and moving every half hour. Or ask your boss for more work to do. You'll get healthier and earn a promotion at the same time!

- Sitting around the house and thinking about munching? Get up and go for a walk, call a friend, clean the house, knit, play a game or instrument or prepare a batch of healthy meals for the week. The best distraction is one that keeps your brain and hands occupied.

PLAN YOUR "CHEAT" MEALS OR DAYS

You are supposed to indulge. I repeat, you are supposed to indulge…that is what keeps us balanced and sane. The key is to control how and when you indulge to get the results you want. From your assessment you can probably tell whether you're the type of person who has a lot of little indulgences, like a cookie here and some French fries there, or a few big indulgences such as three course meal extravaganzas or big drinking nights. Or you may be a bit of both.

A common indulgence mindset I use with people is the "80/20 approach," another brainchild of Amanda Carlson-Phillips, VP of Nutrition and Research for Athletes' Performance and Core Performance. The 80/20 approach involves making healthy decisions 80% of the time, which is four out of every five meals or snacks, because you know that you won't make the healthiest decisions the other 20% of the time either by choice or due to circumstances. Based on your preferences, that can translate into either a small, indulgent snack every day, a moderate indulgent meal a few times a week or a full day of indulgence once a week.

Read through your Indulgence Frequency Assessment and decide which indulgences you truly enjoyed the most. Think about both the food and the circumstances. Then review your daily or weekly schedule and choose how or when you will indulge. By having a plan, you can look forward to indulging on your terms and know that you aren't being restricted from enjoying the foods you love. And if you end up indulging at an unplanned time, you can always adjust your plans to maintain your 80/20 balance.

Those 20% are times for you to choose foods that you like eating, despite knowing that they aren't the healthiest for you. These indulgences are meant to be savored and satisfying. They shouldn't create a sense of guilt, because they're part of your plan and you're intending to eat and enjoy them.

If you find that 80/20 isn't getting you the results you want, you can always kick it up a notch towards 90/10: Eat healthfully at 90% of meals and indulge at the other 10%. Eating healthy 100% of the time is very risky because at that point you're probably restricting yourself. Can you go without a cookie, French fry or burger for the rest of your life? Research shows that feelings of restriction inevitably lead to frustration and an overwhelming urge to eat the foods that you're keeping yourself from enjoying. And when you finally give in, do you just have a little bit of what you wanted? Or do you go overboard? Balance and moderation not only involves eating well, but also enjoying the occasional indulgence.

MAKE SOCIAL EATING HEALTHIER AT RESTAURANTS

Being health conscious can be an uphill battle when eating out, since many restaurant meals are higher in calories than similar, home-cooked versions. For example, imagine making a grilled chicken salad at home. You have some lettuce, mixed vegetables, grilled chicken, a little reduced-fat shredded cheese and some dressing. Assuming a standard, three ounce chicken breast, one ounce of cheese and two tablespoons of dressing, the salad would amount to about 400-450 calories.

On the other hand, as of June 2012, an "Oriental grilled chicken" salad from Applebee's has 1290 calories, almost three times the calories of your homemade salad and over half of an average person's daily calorie requirement! And people may think they're eating healthy when they choose this menu item, because it's a salad. But as you can see, appearances can be deceiving. By the way, I'd like to note that Applebee's and similar restaurants now offer a number of reasonable, lower-calorie options. It's just a matter of finding them highlighted on the menu or asking your waiter.

The difference in calories between the homemade and the restaurant salads is likely due to the restaurant's large portion size and higher-calorie additions, such as croutons and excess amounts of cheese and dressing. To make the salad lower in calories, ask for less cheese, dressing on the side and take half of the salad home for tomorrow's lunch.

Salads aside, most of us will continue to eat out on a regular basis, and few want to spend lots of time sorting through nutrition facts. The following tips will prepare you to make quick, healthy decisions when eating at restaurants – allowing you to enjoy your food without extra calories!

Choosing the restaurant

- Choose restaurants that offer healthy options, such as grilled or broiled meats and fish, and healthy side items, such as fruits and vegetables.
- Avoid buffets. You're more likely to overeat, and you can't take home leftovers for future meals.
- Look for lunch or early bird specials, so you can eat at establishments with healthier options for less money.

Choosing menu items

- Scan the menu for a "lighter," "low-calorie," or "healthy option" section, but then don't let the name fool you; read the menu descriptions.

- Look for words such as baked, roasted, grilled, broiled, steamed, cooked in its own juices, marinara or tomato sauce, choice or select cuts of meat and broth- or tomato-based soups.

- Order items less frequently that use words such as fried, sautéed, batter dipped, breaded, au gratin, scampi, Alfredo, cooked with butter or cream, gravy, prime cuts of meat and cream-based soups.

- A salad is usually a safe bet for a healthy entrée. Just ask for dressing on the side and request reduced amounts of high-calorie add-ons such as cheese, creamy dressings, etc.

- Look at the appetizer menu, which sometimes contains the only healthy options at a restaurant. See if you can mix-and-match an appetizer with a side salad, soup, or a second healthy appetizer.

- If you really want to order a higher-calorie entrée or dessert, ask someone to split it with you so you can enjoy the food while having half the calories.

- When in doubt, opt for simpler dishes, such as baked or broiled chicken, instead of ordering something with a lot of mystery ingredients, such as a casserole, stew, or other mixed dish.

Ordering

- Ask the waiter how items are prepared, and what they're served with.

- Are the vegetables buttered? If so, ask if you can get them steamed with no butter, or on the side.

- Order toast and baked potatoes dry, or with spreads and toppings on the side.

- Substitute salsa, plain yogurt, lemon, vinegar or low-calorie salad dressings for higher-calorie dressings and toppings.

- Tell your waiter to "hold the mayo" and put sauces, salad dressings and other high-fat extras on the side.

- Choose a green side salad, steamed vegetable, baked potato or fruit cup in place of the coleslaw, potato salad or French fries that normally come with a meal. If it costs more, ask yourself: is my health worth a one or two dollar substitution charge?

- Order smaller portions, such as half the rice or a small order of French fries, instead of the standard medium portion that accompanies most meals.

Dining

- Avoid overeating by drinking a tall glass of water before you start eating, and drink several glasses during your meal.

- Request a to-go container immediately when you're served a large portion, and put half away before you start eating—two meals for the price of one. Similarly, when you're eating at home, put leftovers away before you start eating.

- Share a large meal or dessert with someone.

- Ask to have high-calorie dressings, gravies, or creamy sauces served on the side instead of directly on top of your food.

- Enjoy the dressing, gravy, or sauce that you've asked to be served on the side by dipping your fork into it before each bite of entrée—you'll get a taste of the dressing, gravy, or sauce in each bite, but you'll consume much less of it by the end of the meal.

- Ask the waiter to remove your plate as soon as you feel full to prevent picking at it.

- Request that your waiter remove the bread or chip basket, or move it out of your reach yourself, if you feel you're snacking too much.

- Eat slowly, put your fork down between bites and chew well.

- Take deliberate steps to end your meal; brush your teeth, chew gum, or drink a tall glass of water to cue yourself that the meal is over.

- When you're done, ask the waiter to remove your plate promptly or give you a to-go container for any leftovers.

- If you're at a party (technically not a restaurant, but you're still eating out), move away from the food as soon as you're done eating.

REPLACE SOCIAL EATING WITH A SOCIAL ACTIVITY

For many of us, spending time with friends or family means food. Hey, we've gotta eat, right? So why not do it with others? In fact, a relationship-building book was written about it: *Never Eat Alone* by Keith Ferrazzi.

But what are we usually eating when we socialize with others? Salads and smoothies? Or buffet-style pot lucks with a few glasses of wine or beer? Or a three-course dinner at a restaurant? Social eating lends itself to indulgence, and while that's not a bad thing now and then, doing it too often can lead to excess calories and weight gain. For example, one big night out with dinner and drinks for *your* birthday will not ruin your health and weight loss pursuits. One big night out every week for *everyone's* birthday might. That's the difference between an occasional indulgence and an indulgent habit.

Social eaters sometimes feel that making improvements to their eating habits means they can no longer socialize with their friends...because that's what they do together. Being social = eating out or cooking. Food might be the preferred topic of conversation as well, especially for foodies such as me. I would rebel too if I felt that eating healthier required me to never see my friends or family again.

Of course, that's not the case. We can do lots of things with our friends or family that don't revolve around eating. But we haven't been required to think about doing something else in a long time, if ever. And when we stop performing a certain habit, such as social eating, there's a void left to be filled: "So if we're not eating, what do I do with my friends and family?"

If that void is left empty, usually one of two things happens:

1. We stop seeing our friends or family because we can't think of something else to do. Then we get fed up with being unsocial and go back to our old habit of social eating.

2. We try to see our friends or family without an idea of what to do. So after twenty minutes of debate about it, everyone gets fed up and decides to just eat.

So this strategy is devoted to an alternative to social eating: social activity. I'm not asking you to replace all of your social eating with social activity. Just make one substitution per week. If you eat socially three times a week, try two days of social eating and one day of social activity. Here are a few ideas to get you started:

- A game of tennis, racquetball or ping pong
- Shoot pool – drink water or seltzer, not beer
- Charades – you'll be surprised how much you move in that game
- Go for a swim
- A round of golf or mini golf
- Going for a group walk or jog – bring the pets along
- Shoot some hoops
- Go dancing
- Go bowling, without the beer and nachos
- Go to the gym together and motivate each other
- Go rock climbing
- Go hiking

Will it take some effort to learn where you can do these things and get ready for them? Yep, but choosing a restaurant or cooking requires work too, so you're probably not wasting much time. And once you find a good social activity, you can do it over and over again with much less effort. You may find yourselves talking about things besides food, too – such as what hiking trails you like or your latest dance moves.

And the results can be surprisingly effective: A full three-course dinner including appetizer, entrée, dessert and beverage can easily run 1500 to 2000 calories…and even higher if you're the type that prefers steaks and Fettuccini Alfredo. On the other hand, some of the activities listed above can burn any-where from 150 to 400 calories per hour. When you add it up, replacing one social meal with one hour of social activity can be a difference of 1650 to 2500 calories per week, equal to about half a pound or more. Half a pound a week over 52 weeks means 26 less pounds a year; small change, big result. Stay so-cial…just use your legs.

FIGHT UNWANTED TEMPTATIONS AND CRAVINGS

Cravings and temptations to indulge in less healthy foods are real and can be very strong. For some it's the smell of freshly baked cookies, and for others, like me, it's the sight of an ice cream parlor. The pull of these cravings can over-ride whatever else you were thinking or talking about. Remember the last time you smelled your favorite food. Did you immediately stop what you were doing and focus on the food? And then could you not get the food out of your mind until you had some? We can't get our mind off of it. Research has even shown that we can make our bodies hungry by just *imagining* our favorite foods – sorry for making you imagine, just needed to prove a point! So if your food cravings are for something less healthy than broccoli and blueberries, be aware of how your body reacts to temptations and take steps to minimize or eliminate their gravitational pull. Here are a bunch of ideas:

1. *Have a plan* – If you already have a plan for what meals and snacks you're eating that day, you can focus on those foods and anticipate the next meal…rather than thinking about the Snickers bar in the vend-ing machine or the free brownies that someone brought into work that day.

2. *Keep healthy snacks available at all times* – If you have healthy snacks around you at home, at work and with you on-the-go, you can turn to those better options to satisfy your cravings. It can be something as simple as a piece of fruit and a few of your favorite nuts.

3. *Have small, frequent meals* – We tend to be more swayed by cravings when we haven't eaten for a few hours – that's the result of hunger and low blood sugar. Then we give in to our craving, get a sugar high and crash again a few hours later. This food spike and crash can become a vicious cycle. If you just ate a satisfying, healthy snack or meal, though, you're a lot less likely to overindulge in cookies or candy. You might still have one cookie, but probably not half the stack.

4. ***Out of sight, out of mind at home*** – If you know certain foods are sure to tempt you into less healthy decisions, make sure they're not around you. Look through your pantry or fridge at home and trash the junk food that you know you can't eat in moderation – any food that you always end up having the whole box of in one sitting, for example.

5. ***Out of sight, out of mind at work*** – If you have a candy jar on your desk for co-workers or clients, are you actually eating more of it than anyone else? If so, get rid of it. This works with candy jars at home too. If a coworker or boss near you has a candy jar and you find yourself indulging frequently, ask them to take the candy off their desk too. If they won't, see if they'll be willing to put it in an opaque, covered jar – you can even buy them one. You won't think about the candy as much if you can't see it.

6. ***Have a go-to, non-food stress reliever*** – If you use food as a way to make yourself feel better, try experimenting with other methods of dealing with stress such as meditation, prayer, yoga, deep breathing, exercise or any other process that allows you to resolve your stress without taking in unneeded calories.

7. ***Hydrate!*** – Sometimes we eat when we're actually thirsty rather than hungry, because the body is looking to get water any way it can. Drinking a glass or two of water (ice-cold with a squirt of lemon helps if you don't like water) and waiting ten to fifteen minutes will let you know whether your craving was a result of hunger or just thirst. When you give your body the water it needs, the food craving may disappear.

8. ***Stay busy*** – It's common to eat because we're bored and have nothing else to do. This can happen when watching TV at night, sitting in front of a computer screen all day or during downtime at work. Watching less TV, taking up a hobby such as playing the guitar, photography or knitting and asking for more responsibility at work are a few ways to fill in the gap.

9. ***Focus on Why you don't want to give in to the craving*** – This is why

keeping an index card with your Whys in your wallet or purse can be very useful. Every time you feel a craving or temptation, pull out the paper and read the reasons why you want to change your eating habits – and decide whether the food you're craving will help you succeed. Those fifteen seconds can be all the time you need for your craving to subside.

10. *Stay active* – Being physically active helps regulate hunger, especially if you're sitting for long periods of time at work, followed by sitting in front of the TV at home. At work, try to do some stretching, chair squats or downward dogs with your hands on your desk every half hour. Scheduling a few brief, ten- or fifteen-minute walks throughout the day, even just around the parking lot, can go a long way towards preventing cravings and temptations.

11. *Keep track of your indulgences* – This is why you assess your indulgences; the more you're aware of them, the better you can control them. As famous businessman and investor Peter Drucker said, "You can't manage what you don't measure." You could also keep a notepad with you and write down your cravings as they occur. Note what food you're craving, the time of day, what's going on right then in your day – a new deadline at work? – and how you feel – stressed? It may clue you in to what you really need in that moment…is it food, or something else? Force the logical side of your brain to ask, "Do I really want this food, or is there a better option?" Looking back on your assessment and notes can also help you identify cravings that really are physical rather than psychological. On days you skip breakfast, you may notice an 11 AM trip to the vending machine for a pastry. Or perhaps you tend to experience a pre-dinner snack binge if you leave work stressed and hungry from not eating since noon.

12. *Look for patterns and create alternatives* – Do you always feel compelled to have soda with pizza, or chips with a sandwich? What makes you crave these foods? Do you like the fizz of the soda with the pizza

or the crunch of the chips with the sandwich? If you notice a pattern, write down what about the food you crave and a similar, healthier food you can have in its place. For example, you could have a carbonated, fizzy seltzer with the pizza, or crunchy vegetables like carrots, celery or water chestnuts with the sandwich.

EMOTIONAL EATING, PART 1: WHEN FOOD IS A SOURCE OF FEELINGS OR CONTROL

People can have relationships with food that extend far beyond their body's need for fuel:

- *Food & Feelings:* Call it stress eating or emotional eating; people who use food to cope with challenges, changes and feelings will find that the very thing they turn to when times get tough is no longer available to them when they start reducing indulgences.

- *Food & Control:* People who have very hectic or demanding daily routines may view food as the last bit of control that they have in their day. So they will choose what they want…and to hell with what anyone else may want them to do or eat. They rebel with food.

- *Food & Cultural Events:* Sometimes food is the focus of every family or cultural event: parties, weddings, funerals and Sunday dinners. Food becomes a reflection of love and caring. So you're not just eating for yourself, you're eating for those who cooked for you. And unfortunately, if these events are all-day eating bonanzas with a non-stop stream of appetizers, heavy entrées and desserts, you can be eating way more than your body has bargained for.

When you listen to these external cues for eating such as stress and guilt – how can you turn down Grandma's homemade apple pie? – you override your body's natural signals of hunger and fullness. If you repeatedly override these systems, you may end up in a state where you can only feel ravenously starving or exceedingly full rather than just hungry or satisfied. And as you become less able to sense your body's signals, you start relying more and more on your feelings and emotions to dictate your eating habits instead. As Fat Bastard eloquently said in *Austin Powers: The Spy Who Shagged Me*: "I eat because I'm unhappy, and I'm unhappy because I eat."

Food has become a dependency in this case, equally as strong as drugs for addicts, cigarettes for smokers, or booze for alcoholics. Research shows that when people quit smoking, they tend to gain weight. This can be partially attributed to the fact that nicotine is an appetite suppressant, but it's also possible that food becomes the new coping mechanism. When people who smoked used to get stressed, they'd smoke. Now that the cigarettes are no longer there, they need to find a new coping mechanism. While healthy coping mechanisms exist such as exercise, yoga and meditation, food might be the most convenient one. Hence the weight gain.

Also consider this: What is one of the main ingredients in popular comfort foods such as cookies, chocolate, cake and brownies? Carbs, particularly sugar. High doses of sugar can have an impact on the brain similar to cocaine. That's not just theory...sugar and cocaine activate the same dopamine receptors and feel-good chemicals in the brain. But of course, after a while, the effects wear off and we need to look for the next "hit" if we didn't resolve the original source of emotion or stress.

While I'll be the first to admit that this isn't an easy undertaking, the solution for emotional eaters is to find alternate ways to feel in control or cope with stress. Trying to resolve the sources of stress is a great start, and activities later in the book will go over good ways to do this.

Next, it's about finding other stress management activities that you feel comfortable turning to during tough times – especially during challenges you face in the health, fitness or weight change process. Exercise, yoga, meditation, crafts, cooking, calling a friend, and getting more sleep are just a few, but you should figure out what will work for you. Sometimes you just need to review your Whys. When you start turning to activities other than eating to handle stress, you can slowly reclaim your body's natural hunger and fullness systems. And once again you'll be able to eat when you're actually hungry, rather than when you are happy, sad, mad, etc.

EMOTIONAL EATING, PART 2: FIND THE SOURCE OF YOUR INDULGENCES

Are you in control of your indulgences? Do you choose to have them when you want, or eat them because you have a sudden urge and can't say no? Answering these can help you understand the difference between physical and emotional hunger. Adam Gilbert, founder of MyBodyTutor.com, has written an insightful piece on this topic:

"Real, physical hunger comes on gradually. Emotional hunger comes on suddenly. Real hunger can be satisfied with any food. Yes, that's right—if an apple doesn't satisfy our hunger, we're not truly physically hungry.

Emotional hunger, on the other hand, comes with a craving for a specific food. And, unfortunately, it's usually not for apples. Ever have those times when you eat snack after snack and nothing seems to be hitting the spot? Well, that's because you're not physically hungry. You're emotionally hungry.

When we get "hungry" it's worth asking ourselves a few questions:

1. How long has it been since I've eaten?

2. What was the last thing I ate? Was it something nutritious?

3. What am I really hungry for?

4. Is anything bothering me?

5. If I had an 'EASY' button to magically help me with what I'm dealing with, right now, what would I use it for?

Perhaps, what you're hungry for is affection, assistance, rest, excitement, peace of mind. Is it possible to have the need met by someone? How about by yourself? Here's the challenge: Many times we feel like our needs can't or won't get met—so food becomes our escape. When we're "hungry," that is a need we feel like we can actually control.

Sometimes, it can be very helpful to explore what it feels like to have the need go unmet by simply writing about it. Many clients have reported that this eases the discomfort tremendously. This is also how you can find out what you might really want out of your life because typically we'd shovel food into our mouth so we don't have to experience or face the feelings. Because when we're not suppressing feelings, they'll come to the surface, and we'll be able to see what it is we truly want.

Food is only love when it is used to feed our true physical hunger or when we actually enjoy, relish and savor the experience (not feel guilty in the moments afterwards). Otherwise, we're using food to cover up feelings. Feelings that are preventing us from becoming the person we really want to be. How do you like them apples?"

And two more tips from Adam:

1.   Many times we just finish the food in front of us simply because it's, well, in front of us. Try asking yourself this question mid-meal, "Would I eat an apple right now?" If the answer is no, you're not physically hungry anymore. That's why the easiest way to eat less is to serve ourselves less. We can't eat what's not there. And if we serve ourselves less, we don't have to bother asking ourselves questions mid-meal!

2.   When we're faced with an intense craving, we're usually only thinking about that craving. We're not thinking about anything else. And because of that, we can't imagine our life without giving in to those cravings.

Here's the challenge: a lot of people can't imagine what life would be like without having that nighttime dessert. And because we can't imagine our life without our "usual" dessert, we think, "Screw it. Why bother? I deserve this and I'm entitled to this because I work hard." Why do we do this? Because the discomfort in that moment is too great. So we have to rationalize it away.

But this situation can apply to many aspects of life, not just food. Imagine you're a swimmer and your friend is terrified of jumping in the pool. *You* know how much fun it is but she doesn't. Or you know that an amusement park ride is really fun but the person you're with is scared. Or you're eating this weird-looking food that's absolutely delicious. But the person you're with is grossed out, and doesn't want to try it. What would you say? Probably something along the lines of, "Just try it once. Everything will be okay. What's the worst that can happen?"

What I'm suggesting is that if you want to break that after-dinner dessert habit, focus only on not having it today. Don't worry about tomorrow or next week. Just focus on today. Because once we go through the evening without that dessert, we realize it's actually doable, and not nearly as bad as we thought it would be. But again, we can't know that unless we "just jump in" and try it once.

IN CONCLUSION: SUMMARIZE YOUR RELATIONSHIP WITH FOOD

In the end, we're all somewhere along the same continuum. On one end there's Eating to Live, where food is only fuel to you. The other extreme is Living to Eat, where food and cravings are a constant focus in life, from social functions to emotions. The key is striking the balance that allows us to enjoy food when we want while being mindful of and listening to our natural hunger and satiety signals. We choose nourishing, healthy foods whenever we can because we know there will be special occasions when we'll choose not to and instead will indulge and enjoy it. It's not about restriction…it's about balance.

Take a piece of paper and draw a line across it. At one end of the line write "Eat to Live" and on the other end write "Live to Eat." Make a mark on the line where you feel you currently lie on the continuum. The middle of the line would indicate that you equally prioritize "Eating to Live" and "Living to Eat." Next, make a mark where you believe you would need to be on this continuum to get the health, fitness or weight changes you desire and achieve your Whys. Don't worry about the distance between the two marks. Just focus on brainstorming a couple ideas of how you can make one small shift from where you currently are to where you want to be. Remember, the hardest part of any journey is the first step.

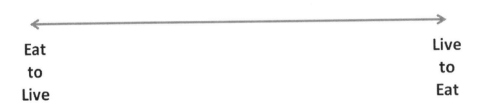

Eat
to
Live

Live
to
Eat

HABIT 6: INCREASE YOUR PHYSICAL ACTIVITY

RATIONALE

The many benefits of being regularly active could probably fill a couple pages on their own. Here's a brief summary:

- Reduces risk of cardiovascular disease, stroke, repeat heart attacks, Type 2 diabetes and some cancers
- Lowers cholesterol, triglycerides, blood pressure
- Improves insulin sensitivity
- Reduces osteoporosis risk
- Allows you to achieve and maintain a healthy body weight by burning calories and boosting your metabolism
- Reduces feelings of stress, anxiety and depression as effectively as anti-depressants
- Builds and maintains healthy bones, muscles and joints
- Helps keep us strong, able and independent as we age, including reducing the risk of falling

These benefits have a "dose-response," which means that people who do little or no activity will significantly improve their health and fitness levels as they start an exercise program. In other words, getting off the couch and exercising even once per week can have a huge impact on your health, fitness and weight: an extra four to ten pounds of weight loss each year. Moderately active people who start working out more often or more intensely will experience smaller, but still very real, improvements to their metabolism, fitness and health levels.

And the benefits of being physically active go beyond fitness and avoiding chronic disease. In psychiatrist Dr. Daniel Amen's book, *Change Your Brain, Change Your Body*, almost every chapter recommends exercise to improve the mind and body, including:

- Reducing food cravings
- More balanced hormones
- Better skin and complexion
- Better focus and energy

- Improved sleep
- Stronger memory
- Less stress
- Increased sex drive

If you'd like to improve any of the issues listed above, consider increasing your physical activity.

For those that are already quite active, imagine having to push against that spring discussed in Chapter 4. If you feel confident that you can consistently add another day of exercise to your routine, then go for it! But if you're already training four days a week, think about whether you could benefit more from another Easy Eight Habit rather than pushing yourself to schedule a fifth workout. If you start training five or more days per week, you'll also need to devote more time and effort toward recovery for your body to avoid injury – that means sleep, proper nutrition, and stretching or foam rolling.

ASSESSMENT

Using the Weekly Physical Activity Tracker, note how much time you spend exercising on a weekly basis. You'll be able to track the day, duration, type and intensity of your exercise. Include any type of planned activity such as running, biking, going to the gym, lifting weights or participating in sports like tennis, golf, basketball games or softball. Also give yourself credit for recreational activities such as hiking, dancing or strenuous household work like cleaning or gardening. Then add up the total number of days and minutes you spent exercising: that's your baseline.

RECOMMENDATION

Based on the number of days and minutes you are currently active, aim to increase your planned physical activity by either thirty minutes of activity or one workout per week. If you have an inconsistent weekly schedule, aim for a monthly goal of either four more workouts or two more hours of activity per month – the weekly goal times four. The strategies section below has plenty of ideas for activities in addition to the ones mentioned earlier. You can choose any activity that gets you moving, sweating and your heart rate up. Just be sure that it's planned and performed on a regular basis!

EASY EIGHT HABIT #6 STRATEGIES

30 WAYS TO INCREASE YOUR PLANNED PHYSICAL ACTIVITY WITHOUT A GYM

1. Go for a walk or run with a friend or your family!

2. Go dancing with a friend or significant other.

3. Walk the golf course rather than taking a cart.

4. Learn a new activity like ice skating or rollerblading.

5. Jump rope.

6. Clean your house or apartment with some elbow grease.

7. Walk to stores that are within half a mile of your home – or more.

8. Play "active" video games like Dance, Dance Revolution or Wii Fit games.

9. Garden! Start a fruit and vegetable patch or a flower bed.

10. Buy a pedometer to track your walking. Works great for number-oriented people.

11. Do bodyweight exercises anywhere, such as squats, lunges, pushups, planks, jogging in place, mountain climbers or jumping jacks.

12. Do some of your own house repairs.

13. Start a walking club at work. Walk ten or fifteen minutes every day around the parking lot or the halls in the morning, during lunch and in the afternoon.

14. Go biking with friends or family, or bike to work.

15. Play Frisbee with some friends.

16. Play active games like ping pong or air hockey, which involve coordination, speed and skill.

17. Do bodyweight exercises at commercial breaks when watching TV; that can be five minutes or more of exercise for every half hour of TV time!

18. Relieve your landscaping service and do your own yard work: save money and get a workout.

19. Build something for your house like a table, desk, shelves or bookcase.

20. Take your dog for more walks or runs.

21. Look for places to be active in your community such as parks, big patches of grass, or basketball, tennis or handball courts.

22. Get an exercise DVD or join a group fitness class—just remember to always listen to yourself physically, not the demands of the instructor. When in doubt, ask.

23. Disconnect the TV: You'll do more active things when you're not tempted to sit for hours in front of the screen. Test it out: Put your cable on hold for one month and see how it goes.

24. Find a local pool and go swimming—great for cardiovascular and resistance training.

25. Join an intramural sports team – would you enjoy volleyball, basketball, tennis, or another sport?

26. Help your friends or family next time they move to a new place.

27. Plan active things to do on vacation, such as walking-based sightseeing, swimming, kayaking, hiking, etc.

28. Go hiking or join a hiking club. Can't find one? Form your own via an existing community organization or via Meetup.com.

29. Teach your friends how to exercise!

30. Make your social time focused on activities like tennis or basketball, rather than eating out.

THE THREE PRINCIPLES OF A SAFE AND EFFECTIVE PHYSICAL ACTIVITY PROGRAM

No matter what activities you choose to increase, it's important to take the necessary steps to maximize results while avoiding injury. Unfortunately, most people are either unaware of or misinformed about these issues. This section has the questions to ask and issues to consider when you develop your exercise or planned physical activity routine. Keep these three key principles in mind:

1. Match the Warm-up to the Demands
2. Work the Whole Body
3. Recover for Results

ONE: MATCH THE WARM-UP TO THE DEMANDS

Why Warm Up?

Some physical actions happen all the time in daily life, like standing up, picking things up, walking, turning, reaching, etc. Your brain is going to make your body do them regardless of whether or not you use the right muscles and joints. When the right muscles and joints are not available due to chronic muscle tightness, the brain compensates and asks other muscles and joints to pick up the slack and get the job done. Unfortunately, these "backup" muscles and joints are the ones that become painful and injured. As Charlie Weingroff puts it, "It's the victim that cries, not the perpetrator!" A classic example is pain in the lower back or knee (victim) due to tightness in the hip (perpetrator), caused by sitting all day.

These issues are often due to the constant positions we hold and the repetitive motions we perform on a daily basis. Do you sit most of the day? Do you hunch or lean forward at your desk to read a computer screen? Or are you on your feet for many hours? Do you have to turn, move or lift repeatedly throughout the day? Do you carry your bag, backpack, briefcase or groceries on the same side regularly? Do you frequently wear high heels? These are all potential contributing factors to movement compensations and increased injury risk.

Now imagine doing workouts with these movement compensations. If you add weight to poor movement patterns, you are building a house on a shaky foundation. Odds are, the more we build, the more stress we'll place on that faulty foundation until it cracks and collapses—along with the house. You need a solid foundation of healthy movement patterns without compensations before adding significant weight and intensity to your movements. Otherwise you'll reinforce these poor movements and drive yourself to injury even faster. That's why you can get injured if you do too much too fast; your body isn't prepared to handle that intensity.

A warm-up helps restore healthy movement patterns and prepares your brain and body for the upcoming workout or physical activity. You'll get the most out of your workouts this way – moving better, farther and harder – while minimizing your risk of injury.

A lot of people warm up by running on a treadmill or cycling on a bike for five minutes to break a light sweat and "get warm." While this does help raise core temperature and loosen up some joints, it's often inadequate. Whatever you choose to do, know that an effective warm-up must do two things:

1. Release any tight muscles to prevent putting strain on the wrong joints or ligaments when training, which is a major cause of chronic pain and injury.
2. Get all of the target muscles and joints "awake" and engaged before you start your physical activity or workout.

To accomplish this, focus on the three components of an effective warm-up: myofascial release, dynamic or active stretching and movement preparation.

Myofascial Release

The best example of myofascial release is massage therapy, particularly deep tissue or sports massage. The massage therapist uses their hands to find tight "trigger points" within the muscle and release them. Releasing these knots, trigger points or adhesions can be uncomfortable, but you should feel a ton better afterward. You feel looser, more relaxed and notice that you can move more freely. Yet within a few days the tightness returns—usually due to the fact that you continue to do the same movements and postures that got you tight to begin with. So you could go back to the massage therapist. But we don't all have the time or money to see a massage therapist on a regular basis. Enter self-myofascial release!

In many ways, self-myofascial release is a lighter version of massage therapy. While nothing can fully replace the precision and depth of a pair of human thumbs (or elbows), applying pressure on an overworked or stiff muscle's trigger points using items like a foam roller (pictures of that coming up), pinky ball, tennis ball, frozen water bottle, softball or golf ball can bring increased range of motion to joints, more blood flow to the tight muscle and better movement patterns.

These are very similar to the results you'd get from a massage therapist. And if you perform self-myofascial release consistently – at least three times a week for five to fifteen minutes – on your chronically tight muscles, you will likely experience:

1. Reduced risk of injuries while exercising

2. More effective workouts and better athletic performance

3. Less nagging discomfort when performing daily activities

So by now I'm sure you want to know what muscles you need to foam roll and how to do it! The muscles you need to roll, or release, are the chronically tight muscles—and those depend on the positions you hold or movements you do repeatedly. For many people, especially those that sit and hunch forward regularly, five typically tight areas are: the side of the leg (IT Band), the inner thigh, the front of the leg and hip (hip flexors), the chest and the upper back and shoulders area.

Self-myofascial release is a calculated seek-and-destroy mission. Make sure you're rolling on your muscles, not directly over any joints or on bones. As you move the foam roller or tennis ball along the target muscle, you will likely find a particular area that is very uncomfortable. That's an adhesion or trigger point. The key is to apply sustained but not unbearable pressure on that area, breathe, and relax the muscle onto the ball or roller. Within fifteen to thirty seconds the discomfort will usually begin to dissipate. Once the discomfort is about 75% gone, go on to roll the rest of the muscle. When you come across one trigger point, though, many others may be right around it – so you probably won't have to go very far to find another trigger point. Continue for as long as you feel comfortable; try to get up and down the muscle(s) at least twice. It should get easier the more often you do it.

If you have any acute or chronic joint conditions such as osteoarthritis, rheumatoid arthritis or tendonitis, check with your physician or physical therapist before starting a self-myofascial release program. Other points of concern: be careful if lying on the ground is challenging for you or resting your body weight on the foam roller is too intense – you can adjust how much pressure you apply by leaning against a wall with the foam roller or tennis ball on the target muscle. If you have any concerns about performing these techniques, you should consult a qualified fitness professional to make sure you're doing the movements correctly. Ask the person: "Can you help me with self-myofascial release/foam rolling to help with a tight (name your stiff muscles here)?" If you get a confused look in return, keep looking for a professional who understands your needs!

Here are a few examples of self-myofascial release for different areas of the body:

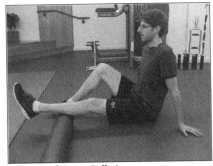
Calves (with Foam Roller)

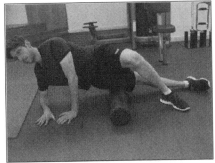
Side of Leg / IT Band (with Foam Roller)

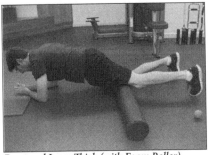
Front and Inner Thigh (with Foam Roller)

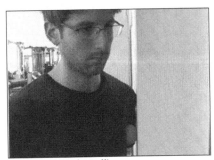
Chest (with Pinky Ball)

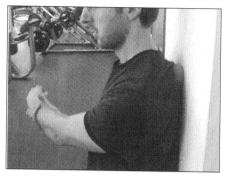
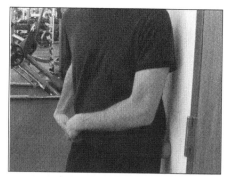

Back and Shoulder (with Pinky Ball)　　　*Hip and Butt/Glute (with Pinky Ball)*

Stretching

Stretching a few times per day, especially if you have to be in the same position all day is a great way to reduce joint discomfort and fight muscle imbalances – for example, you can stretch your calves if you wear heels all day, stretch your hip flexors if you sit, etc. When you're preparing for exercise, though, certain types of stretching are better than others. Here are the main types, along with when they are most appropriate:

Static Stretching – Holding a stretch for an extended period of time until you feel a relaxation in the stretched muscle, about fifteen to thirty seconds. For example, a static stretch for the chest involves making an "L" or "goalpost" with one of your arms, placing it against a doorframe and lightly leaning forward. Several static stretches are shown in the *Recover for Results* section later.

Static stretching has been a controversial topic in the fitness industry recently, particularly regarding whether it's safe to do before a workout. Static stretching tells the stretched muscle to relax. This is a great type of stretch for chronically tight muscles like the hip flexors, chest and calves for people who sit all day. However, when you ask these muscles to relax, you can't then immediately ask them to do the opposite – contract, through exercise – or you're sending mixed messages and increasing injury risk. If you do any static stretching before exercise, do some warm-up exercises before the workout to re-activate those now stretched – but much better aligned – muscles. For example, a slow march in place for a few seconds is a great movement to do after a static hip flexor or quadriceps stretch.

On the other hand, static stretching is great in the middle of a long work-day, when you've been sitting in front of a computer for hours and want to get out of your chair and stretch your hips and chest. You'll promote blood flow to those areas, help prevent movement compensations and just generally feel better when you sit back down. Try doing static stretches at least once an hour if you normally sit for an extended period of time during the day.

Active/Dynamic Stretching – Dynamic stretching, or active stretching as it's also called, is a great way to prepare your body for exercise and movement without having to worry about relaxing your muscles too much as with static stretching. With dynamic stretching, you move your tight muscles through their entire range of motion in a slow, controlled manner for three to six seconds, and repeat that movement a few times. This allows tight muscles to continue to loosen up after self-myofascial release, and helps "turn on" any weaker muscles prior to exercise. Here are a few examples:

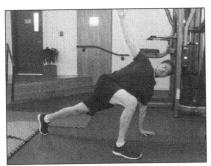
Spiderman Lunge with T-Turn

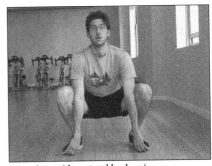
Drop Squat (then stand back up)

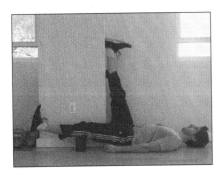
Leg Lowering (and then back up)

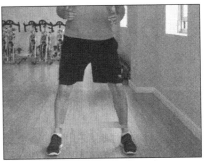
Lateral Mini Band Drill (push with the hip of the trailing leg, don't pull with the lead leg. Go both ways)

Ballistic Stretching – A more explosive type of stretch. Rather than moving slowly through the stretch, like dynamic stretching, ballistic stretching minimizes the time between moving one way and the other to a second or less. This type of stretch includes bouncing up and down on your feet or toes as when jumping rope, swinging your arms forward, backward and in a circle or swinging your leg back and forth. These stretches are designed for people who'll be performing high-intensity activity.

Moving your muscles quickly through their entire range of motion with little to no pause makes it harder for you to control exactly which muscles are moving, unless you're very experienced. Because of this, people who are new to exercise are more likely to be injured doing this type of stretch. If you choose to do ballistic stretching, do other warm-ups first, like myofascial release and/ or dynamic stretching.

Proprioceptive Neuromuscular Facilitation (PNF) Stretching – This is an advanced version of static and dynamic stretching, in which you temporarily contract the stretched muscle to get it to relax further once you stretch it again. Here's the sequence for PNF stretching:

1. Stretch the target muscle with 10 seconds of static stretching.

2. While holding the same position, engage the target muscle for 6 seconds.

3. Re-relax and statically stretch the target muscle for another 10-20 seconds.

You should notice that by contracting and then re-releasing the target muscle, you'll be able to stretch the muscle more deeply. As this is an advanced movement, I recommend discussing it with a qualified fitness professional if you're unsure of the technique.

Movement Preparation: Getting Your Muscles and Joints Ready for Physical Activity

Movement preparation exercises mimic the joint motions that you'll perform during your planned physical activity. If you're getting ready to play baseball, choose warm-ups that will prepare you to do the movements involved in that sport. For example, you should prepare the shoulder for throwing and swinging, and prepare the hips and ankles for running, lunging and possibly diving. Just about everyone needs to prepare the core, or trunk, for movement before exercising – this keeps your lower back safe from injury. Classic exercises for the core are the plank or side plank.

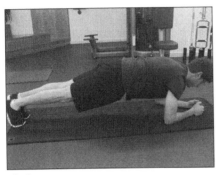

Plank

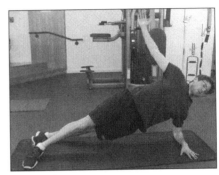

Side Plank

So, if you're about to play a sport or do an activity, think about the movements you'll be performing and what joints are active in those movements :

- Will you be turning repeatedly when dancing?
- Will you be jumping or running when playing basketball?
- Will you be squatting or lunging when gardening?
- Will you be turning, reaching or swinging when playing tennis or golf?

The simplest way to come up with movement preparation exercises is to, in fact, do a less intense version of the exercise you are about to do. If you're going to do bench presses, for example, do a lighter set first. Dynamic stretches are also great for movement preparation. You can eventually move up to more progressive exercises such as bodyweight squats, lunges and jumping jacks.

If you're just getting into physical activity, movement preparation can be a resistance workout on its own—and that's totally fine. In fact, movement preparation inherently contains many of the components of an effective workout plan —because movement preparation is getting your body ready for a workout!

TWO: WORK THE WHOLE BODY

The best workouts engage the entire body. And I'm not just talking about muscles…don't forget your heart, brain, bones and more. To train all of these different parts of the body, keep these four key physical activity components in mind:

1. Engage the trunk, also known as the core
2. Train your brain
3. Move your body against resistance
4. Work the heart and lungs – the cardiorespiratory system

Some sports and activities already include all of these. Take basketball. You need coordination and trunk stability to move smoothly, pass and shoot. You need stamina – which is cardiorespiratory ability – to run up and down the court all four quarters. And you get resistance training from launching your body weight when you jump for shots and rebounds.

Engage the Trunk (aka the Core)

If you have any shoulder, back, hip or knee issues, trunk stability should be of the utmost concern. If you don't have any issues but care about the long-term health of these joints, you should also pay attention.

First, what's the difference between the trunk and the core? The core is usually limited to just the abdominals and the pelvic floor. While these are certainly great areas to focus on, it's a limited view of the muscles involved in true "core stability." True stability and safe movement rely on proper movement across all of the joints from the shoulders to the hips. The shoulder blades need to be stable as your shoulder moves. Your lower back needs to be stable as your hips and upper back move. The problem is that very often our powerful, mobile muscles such as the pecs (chest), deltoids (shoulders) and quads (front thighs) overpower our small but important stabilizing muscles, such as the mid and lower traps (back), abdominals and glutes (rear and side butt muscles). While you may be working some of these smaller muscles, you might not be training them in ways that teaches them how to stabilize.

Consider crunches and sit-ups, two of the least beneficial abdominal exercises in existence. In fact, some of the work of well-respected spine researcher Stuart McGill focuses on how the way most people do crunches and sit-ups may just be making their back problems worse. Think about what you do all day when you're seated at a desk—you're sitting and crunched forward! So why do you need to encourage a position you're locked into every day? In fact, the abdominals, which are actually many different muscle groups working together, are not designed to crunch; they're designed to stabilize the lower back and trunk as you move.

A good trunk stability exercise involves engaging the abs to keep your body steady against a force. The classic example of trunk stabilization is a pushup or plank. When you're moving down in a pushup or holding the top of a plank, gravity is trying to pull your body down towards the earth. Your trunk and abs are the muscles firing to keep you from falling! Too often I see horrible pushup or plank form, because people are using their shoulder muscles instead – and their entire trunk is a wet noodle, collapsing towards the ground. You can tell who these people are—it looks like they're humping the ground. Don't be one of these people. Once you can achieve good plank form using your trunk muscles, you can make the exercise progressively more challenging by adding limb movements such as mountain climbers, jackknives or shoulder walkouts. If planking on your toes is too challenging, you can plank with both your knees and toes on the ground.

So, why is trunk stability important? Not only does it protect your lower back, it also helps maintain other joints including the shoulder, hip and knee. In fact, studies have shown that people with poor trunk stability get injured more often. And this becomes a downward spiral, as research also shows that injuries or pain impair trunk stability.

Unfortunately, sitting all day, driving, hunching over at work and similar daily activities can turn your trunk muscles off – and they usually stay off unless you consciously engage them. If you exercise with these stabilizing muscles disengaged, you're more likely to use the wrong muscles and place stress on the wrong joints when training. Here are some examples of where you should feel, and not feel, some common exercises:

- **Pushups or bench presses:** You shouldn't feel these deep in the shoulder or on the sides of the arm. Chest exercises should be felt in the chest!

- **Same goes for any sort of row:** You should feel it in between the shoulder blades – the exact opposite of the chest – not deep in the shoulder or radiating down the arm.

- **Lying glute bridges:** You should feel it in the butt muscles, not the lower back.

- **Squats or lunges:** You should feel these predominantly in the butt muscles and just a little bit in the front of the leg – the quads. Not the other way around.

So what to do? Focus on exercises that re-engage the trunk stabilizers: the muscles underneath the armpits, in the mid-back, in the classic abs area and in your butt. The example movements below engage all three components of the trunk: downward shrugs for the shoulder blade complex, dead bugs for the abdominal complex and glute bridges for the hip complex:

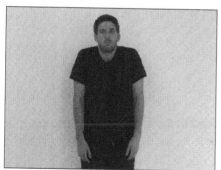
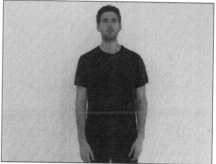

Shoulder Shrug Part 1 of 2: Slowly raise your shoulders up as high as they can go. Raise them gradually as you breathe in and count to four.

Shoulder Shrug Part 2 of 2: Slowly drive your shoulders down, as far down as they can go, while staying steady through the rest of your torso and head. Lower them gradually as you breathe out and count to four. Aim to feel the muscles underneath your armpits engage as the shoulders move down. Those muscles underneath your armpits are your scapular stabilizers and should be working to protect your shoulders when you train.

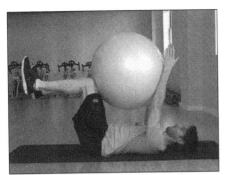

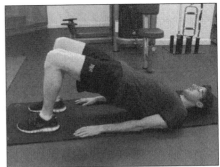

Dead Bugs (with Stability Ball). Do not over-arch your lower back. You can move limbs to make it harder.

Bridges – Raise and lower your butt using your glutes. Keep abs on. You should not feel it in the lower back.

Train Your Brain

A fancy term for training your brain is neuromuscular training. Neuro-muscular means the conversation going on between your brain and muscles; your brain is involved in every movement you perform. If you start doing movements with proper form, your brain will actually create new connections reinforcing that good form – which will make you healthier, stronger and possibly even smarter! And this works for people at any age.

On the other hand, the brain remembers poor movement as well. That's why correct movement patterns are essential. You can promote proper movement patterns by using myofascial release, warming up and learning new exercises properly. Poor form can also creep into your workout when your muscles are fatigued. To avoid that, stop the set and rest when you start to lose good form – don't force out poorly-performed repetitions just because you could do them. Odds are those last reps will be working the wrong muscles, improperly stressing joints and teaching your brain poor movement patterns.

The best known example of neuromuscular exercise is balance training. A simple but effective test of balance is standing on one leg. Keep the knee of the standing leg slightly relaxed. If that's easy, you can spread your arms out and alternate touching your nose with each finger (yes, like they do to see if you are drunk—drinking impacts the neuromuscular system!). If that's easy, try closing your eyes while standing on one leg. And finally if that's easy, try touching your nose with each finger while on one foot with your eyes closed.

Closing your eyes makes balancing much harder because your brain is getting less information about your body's position in space. Also, that's why it's usually easier to balance on one leg by staring at a single point in space or on the ground a few feet away from you.

The goal of neuromuscular training is to make your body get used to staying stable during new movements. Anything that makes you feel a little off-balance or weird is fine…just no pain! Examples of neuromuscular training include:

- Learning a new type of dance.

- Learning a new sport, such as ice skating.

- Doing exercises on one leg, or balancing on one leg.

- Doing unilateral exercises – that is, exercises with just one side at a time. You'll be amazed how much harder doing a chest press is with just one dumbbell—you'll feel your abs turn on like a light bulb. Unilateral exercises can also help improve any imbalances or weaknesses in your body since you tend to be stronger on your dominant hand side.

Move Your Body Against Resistance

Resistance training isn't just lifting weights; it can be any type of activity that makes your muscles work against a resistance. Resistance bands, soup cans, kettlebells, dumbbells or your own body weight are all great forms of resistance training. Yoga, Pilates and swimming can also have an element of resistance training, depending on the intensity and your level of experience. If the exercise has become easy, then you're probably not getting the same benefits you once did.

When lifting weights, beginners should use a weight at which they can do ten to fifteen repetitions *in good form*, with a couple reps "left in the tank." Too often I see people pick up a three pound weight, do fifteen biceps curls and say they did resistance training, although they probably could have done at least twenty more curls without losing form. With the right weight you'll be working hard by the end of your target repetition count. But don't work the muscle until it's jelly, because most people lose form before their muscles completely fatigue. Go for "form failure": the maximum number of repetitions you can do in good form.

Free weights and body weight exercises are ideal because they naturally work your stabilizing muscles by allowing for greater freedom of movement. However, they tend to require more knowledge of how to move safely and properly. This is where training with a fitness professional, even for a couple of months, can be very beneficial. Exercise machines may be a better option than free weights or body weight if you're learning to resistance train on your own, or if you're not able to move your own bodyweight safely. Just make sure you know how to set and use the machine correctly. An improperly set machine can do more harm than good.

When you're ready to increase the challenge, keep in mind that making resistance training more difficult doesn't always mean "more weight is better." Increasing weight is fine to a point, but another great way to progress yourself is to try different movements with the same joints. Your body moves in three planes of motion: sagittal (forward and backward), frontal (side-to-side) and transverse (rotation). Doing an exercise in each plane of motion creates different resistances on your body, engages muscles in different ways and prepares you better for the variety of movements you make in daily life. For example, once you can do basic lunges in good form, you can work up to a series of lunge-based exercises to improve your strength without carrying more weight: reverse and forward lunges for sagittal movement, side lunges for frontal movement, crossover lunges for both frontal and transverse movement, and transverse lunges for...you guessed it...transverse movement.

When in doubt, ask for help! Many gyms have floor trainers who're there to help you learn a new exercise or adjust the machines the first time you use them. But please respect the other people who need their help, and don't keep them occupied for an hour. If you want a private trainer, buy a training session or two.

In fact, if you're new to resistance training, I highly recommend getting expert guidance from a fitness professional with a national certification, preferably from the NSCA, NASM, ACSM or ACE. It's also important to speak with any potential trainer about your goals and make sure they are *listening* to you. They should be focusing on your desired results – not on their idea of what results are. But for brand standards, I would go with the certifications listed above.

Work the Cardiorespiratory System

Cardiorespiratory exercise, often referred to as "cardio," makes your body more efficient at getting oxygen to and through your working muscles. This type of training results in better lung capacity, a stronger heart and more efficient use of oxygen in muscles.

Cardiovascular work typically starts with two to three minutes of continuous, rhythmic movement of large muscle groups. That's why most cardio involves the legs—they house many of your largest muscle groups. Traditional cardio includes walking, running, biking, or using the elliptical or stair climber—anything that you enjoy. Many people are happy to hop on their preferred cardio equipment and watch TV while they do their cardio for 30, 45 or 60 minutes. Others love the feeling of a great, long run outside all across town.

A note on running: Many people love running, and some can do it for their entire lives without issues. Unfortunately, they're the minority. I've worked with countless people who got into running, hit it full throttle and then had to stop within six months because of issues like shin splints, knee pain, back pain and plantar fasciitis. If you intend to take up running for cardio, I highly recommend you get your running form checked out by a gait analysis specialist. Sometimes you can find them at higher-end running shoe stores, but be careful, because they might just be trying to sell you a pair of shoes. Fitness professionals and physical therapists can specialize in running and gait analysis as well, so ask around. Also, you can ask friends who are serious runners who they get coaching from—word of mouth is a great resource. If you live in the New York City area, I recommend my colleagues at the Sports Rehab and Performance Center at Hospital for Special Surgery.

Here are a few tips that can make cardiovascular training more enjoyable and effective:

- *Pay attention to form:* Yes, it's possible to have sloppy form even on a cardio machine – think hunched forward bodies, craning necks and torsos flopping side-to-side. The key to good movement is a stable trunk! Focus on keeping your torso long and your abs engaged as you move your legs or arms. The movement may feel harder, but it'll probably feel better too. Your body will adjust within a few sessions, and then you'll probably see improved ability and improved results.

- *Try a new machine for variety and to challenge the brain.* Some of my favorite cardio machines that can get the job done quickly are the row machine – C2 concepts is a common brand – and the Versa Climber, as they engage both the upper body and the lower body together. Or try a new pattern on a machine you already use. For example, if you usually do the elliptical forwards, try going backwards for a few minutes. Just be sure you have good form.

- *Add periods of increased intensity.* For example, if you like to run for 30 minutes at 6 miles per hour after warming up, try running the first two minutes at 5.5 miles per hour, six minutes at 6 miles per hour, one minute at 6.5 miles per hour and one minute at 7 miles per hour. That's ten minutes. Repeat that three times for a total of thirty minutes. This repeated, gradual increase in intensity is a great way to prepare for interval training, which will get you a cardiovascular response in less time. See below for more details.

Advanced Cardiorespiratory Training: Intervals

Interval training is an advanced, highly effective form of cardio training. It involves brief bursts of higher-intensity work – anywhere from 15 to 60 seconds – followed by a recovery period. A classic example is to run or walk quickly for 30 seconds, then walk more slowly for 60 seconds, and repeat. The amount of time spent resting between high-intensity bursts usually starts at two or three times the length of the burst, like in the example above, but advanced exercisers can reduce rest periods until they're equal to or even shorter than the work phase. Studies have shown that these brief bursts of activity boost your metabolism and may burn more total fat than the "low and slow" cardio that most people consider to be aerobic exercise—and it's over faster! On top of that, interval training can provide many of the same benefits as resistance and neuromuscular training.

Interval training allows you to get more done in less time. The typical interval training workout is no more than 20-25 minutes, plus a warm-up and recovery. You can use most cardio machines and even some lighter resistance training exercises for interval training, including bodyweight exercises, elliptical, running, jump rope or biking.

You can find the right interval intensity for your body with a heart rate monitor, although this requires specialized equipment and a cardiovascular assessment. A less high-tech, but effective alternative is a rating of perceived exertion (RPE). Use RPE to estimate how hard you're working, and progress yourself gradually. This is how it works:

Imagine a scale of 1 to 10, where 1 is the easiest activity ever and you could do it forever. 10 is the hardest, most challenging intensity and you feel like you're going to collapse. After myofascial release and movement preparation, an interval training warm-up period should have you around a 4 to 5. When you get into the interval, you should be pushing yourself anywhere from a 6 to a 9, depending on your experience with training and intervals. Even if you're experienced with exercise, keep in mind that interval training is a new stress on the body, so it may take some time to adapt. Then recover at a rate of about 3 – easier than the warm-up. Repeat this anywhere from six to twelve times, depending on the duration of your interval. For example, a 1-minute "on" and 2-minute "off" interval can be done six times in 18 minutes, while a 30-second "on" and 60-second "off" is performed twelve times in the same period.

As you increase intensity and/or decrease rest time, the harder it will be and the fewer times you'll be able to perform the intervals. And that is totally fine. In fact, one of the most intense forms of interval training, Tabata training, only lasts four minutes! In one study of Tabata training, experienced cyclists performed 20-second all-out bike sprints followed by 10 seconds of slow recovery and repeated that eight times. A number of them couldn't finish the four minutes. Intensity of movement plays a huge role in your body's ability to recover and improve.

Also, when progressing yourself, change only one variable at a time. For example, don't increase intensity via RPE or interval length and also decrease rest time on the same day. I often give clients a little more rest time on days when I progress their intensity. Then we focus on reducing rest time in future sessions.

The key to interval training is pushing yourself in *good form* for a brief period. I cannot express how paramount proper movement is when performing interval training. Don't do interval training on exercises or cardio machines that are new to you. Learn the correct form for any exercise before you push the intensity level. Remember, body weight and non-gym exercises are fine for interval training, so you can do it anywhere—at home or on the road.

A few more interval training tips:

1. ***Focus more on quality than quantity:*** Slowly work up to no more than three interval training sessions per week and supplement with other forms of activity. Too much keeps your body from recovering properly and increases your injury risk.

2. ***Work stronger, not longer:*** A good interval session doesn't have to last longer than 20-30 minutes, plus warm-up and recovery, to get some amazing results. And the greater the intensity of your intervals, the fewer you'll have to do – your body probably won't let you do more anyway.

3. ***Push yourself mentally but listen to yourself physically:*** During interval training our adrenaline is high and we want to do our best. Unfortunately this can also mask injuries and strains, so listen to your body—if something doesn't feel right or you experience a burn in an area where you shouldn't, stop. Try to correct it on the next interval, but if you still feel it, stop, foam roll and recover. Better to stop early one day than to be forced to stop for a few weeks to nurse an injury.

THREE: RECOVER FOR RESULTS

Here's a great rule of thumb I heard from my colleague Antonio Cordova, owner of Precision Athlete in New York City: "The more intense the activity, the more intense the recovery." Good recovery has three components:

1. Myofascial Release & Stretching

2. Recovery Nutrition

3. Rest & Sleep

Myofascial Release and Stretching

Not only do stretching and self-myofascial release work wonders for warm-ups, they also promote recovery by releasing the muscles that are tight from your workout. It's very difficult to foam roll too much. Ideally foam rolling wouldn't hurt anywhere, because that would indicate you have no more adhesions or trigger points. A fantastic goal, but almost impossible, because we're always moving and creating new adhesions. But keep trying!

Static stretching after a good workout is fine, particularly for your chronically tight muscles and the muscles you just exercised. You only need to stretch each muscle for 20 to 30 seconds, so you can do six to eight stretches on both sides of your body within seven to ten minutes. Make sure you have good static stretching form: support the limb you're stretching, and only stretch to mild discomfort—no pain! Here are some chronically tight areas that you can stretch at the end of a workout:

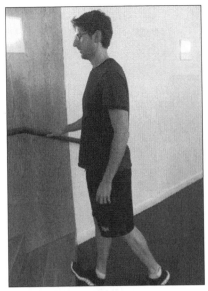

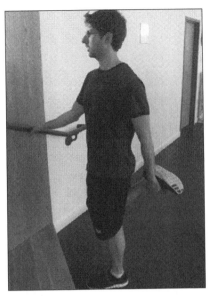

Calves - Do with Straight and then with Slightly Bent Knee

Quadriceps/Front Thigh - Side View

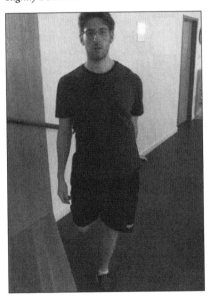

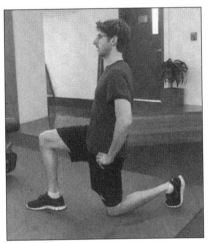

Quadriceps/Front Thigh - Front View

Hip Flexors (Stretches the front of the back leg). You can place the knee on a padded surface. Get tall through spine, tuck back toe in (can un-tuck if knee hurts), tuck tailbone slightly. Stay tall and maintain 90 degree angle in each leg.

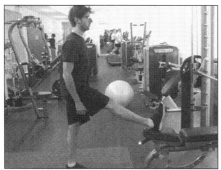

Hamstring - Leg straight and shift hips backward with a straight torso. You don't have to move far.

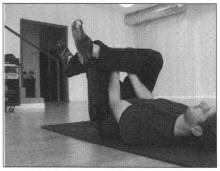

Butt Muscles Stretch (Piriformis, Glutes, etc.). Crossed leg is the stretching leg. Support stretching leg from underneath with hands. Other leg can pull stretching leg towards you further or can stay on the ground with knee bent if you are very tight.

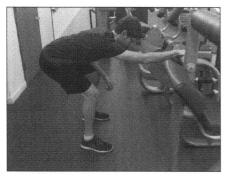

Side of the Trunk - Move back slowly. You should feel this on the side of the torso, not deep in the shoulder.

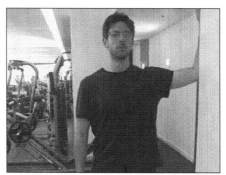

Chest - Starting Position (Elbow around shoulder height, adjust up or down for optimal stretch)

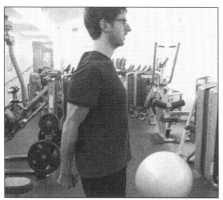

Shoulders - Clasp hands behind back, draw shoulder blades down and back. Don't lean back. Aim for stretch in front/top of shoulders without pain.

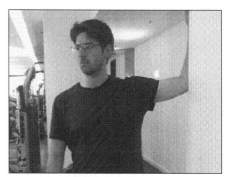

Chest - End Position, Slight Rotation of Trunk. Stretch is felt in chest, not deep in the shoulder or neck.

Ideally you would stretch most, if not all, of your muscles after each workout. If you are pressed for time, stretch your tightest and most worked muscles first. Then get the rest of the muscles in when you can. In other words, if you did running for your activity and you don't have a lot of time to stretch, focus on stretching the legs and chest.

Recovery Nutrition

To exercise consistently, your body needs to be ready for the next workout. What you eat in the hours following physical activity can significantly impact how well and how quickly your body is ready for more activity. While a whole chapter can be devoted to just this topic, here are the nuts and bolts of ideal workout recovery nutrition:

1. This is the time your body is most able to use carbohydrates to replenish fuel stores, so carbs are an important part of post-workout nutrition.

2. Protein is also vitally important after physical activity to give your muscles the building blocks they need to get stronger. Most people need about 15 to 25 grams of protein after a good workout or sports session.

3. Eat your post-workout snack or meal within an hour – preferably within 30 to 45 minutes – of the workout.

4. Athletes, weekend warriors training for a marathon or triathlon and those looking to gain weight require about a three- or four-to-one (3-4:1) carbohydrate-to-protein ratio. So the nutrient label of a good recovery food or drink will have about 45 to 100 grams of carbohydrates in addition to the 15 to 25 grams of protein. This results in a post-workout meal or snack of about 240 to 500 calories.

5. People doing lighter activities or those looking to lose weight may do better with a one-to-one or two-to-one carbohydrate-to-protein ratio. Look for about 15 to 50 grams of carbohydrates in addition to the 15 to 25 grams of protein. That results in a post-workout meal or snack of about 120 to 300 calories.

6. Recovery meals and snacks can be whole foods, or if need be, meal replacement shakes or bars. Athletes and those looking to gain weight can usually just eat *more* of the same healthy foods as those looking to lose weight. Here are some great post-workout mini-meals:

- Low-fat chocolate milk
- Smoothies with fruit, yogurt, milk or whey. Feel free to use a non-dairy protein source as well, such as soy, hemp, peas, etc.
- Fruit and a piece of low-fat string cheese
- Half a sandwich with lean protein
- Small bowl of whole-grain cereal with low-fat milk
- Low-fat yogurt with fruit
- Half a peanut butter sandwich on whole grain bread
- Whole-food-based meal replacements or shakes

If you don't want to add an extra, post-workout meal to your daily routine, work out at a time in the day when your next scheduled meal will be coming up within an hour of finishing your exercise.

Rest & Sleep

Your muscles need anywhere from 24 to 72 hours to recover from a bout of exercise. You need more recovery if you're either new to training or have recently increased your intensity. Believe it or not, your body is actually getting stronger and better when it's recovering after a workout, not during the workout itself.

One of the most common reasons for injury is "too much, too soon." People will work out day after day, week after week without giving their bodies the rest it needs to recover. This can lead to overtraining, which is a clinical condition represented by losing strength, excess fatigue throughout the day and a loss of motivation to be active. In other words, your body is wiped out! If you're just getting off the couch, exercise just once or twice per week for the first few weeks so your body can adapt to the increased activity and so you can make physical activity a real habit in your life—not just an unsustainable burst.

Another thing to keep in mind is that only the muscles that were working really require rest. So full body workouts are best for those of you who are exercising three or fewer times per week, since you'll get about 48 hours of rest between each workout. For those who are more advanced and have more time to devote to resistance training, you can do push/pull or upper/lower body "splits" that allow you to work your body in successive days. For example, you can do upper body exercises such as pushups, rows, shoulder presses and pull-ups one day followed by lower body exercises like squats, lunges, jump rope and leg curls the next day. This allows your upper body to rest at least one full day. These splits are advanced progressions and place joints under a significant load, so they're not a good fit for people who are new to training.

Of course, you don't have to be totally sedentary on your recovery days. Recovery can include some time spent foam rolling, stretching, performing warm-up exercises and even a little bit of light cardio to promote blood flow. Just keep in mind that these extra days are for recovery, not intense training, so you should finish up feeling refreshed and less sore, not more wiped out!

TIPS TO MAXIMIZE PERFORMANCE AND MINIMIZE INJURY RISK

Control the Entire Movement – When you're lifting weights, control the weight at all points in time, even as you move the weight back to the starting position – and especially if your own body is the weight. Otherwise you may place excess strain on your joints and ligaments, which can eventually lead to injury. Focus on a gradual exhale over two to three seconds as you move the weight, and then a gradual inhale over two to three seconds as you return the weight to its starting position. Even the fastest movements must be controlled by going slower at first.

Push Yourself Mentally – Our own thoughts are often what make us stop a few reps short or a few minutes early from what we can really accomplish. Create a positive, supportive environment to make sure you get going, and then do all you can to keep yourself feeling "pumped" during exercise. Listen to inspiring music, actually tell yourself that you *can* do that extra set, close your eyes and visualize that last sprint right before you do it. Elite athletes use these tactics to get the most out of themselves – why not do the same to maximize the benefits of your workouts?

Listen to Your Body Physically – This is the counterpoint to pushing yourself mentally. When we psych ourselves up to go the extra mile, we need to do so safely. We tend to disregard small twinges and tweaks of discomfort when working out. Unfortunately, the adrenaline running through your body during exercise can keep you from feeling pain, and thereby hide a serious issue. "Pushing through it" often leads to even further problems. It's better to stop a little short on a workout because of an unusual twinge than to be forced to stop for weeks because of an injury that you could have prevented by listening to your body.

A personal case-in-point: I remember pushing myself to do farmer's walks, which means walking around with two heavy weights, with two 75-pound dumbbells at the end of a workout. A great trunk stability exercise when performed properly. But I'd already done power hang cleans, a big powerful movement that works similar muscles to the farmer's walk. I felt a slight twinge in my upper shoulder during the farmer's walks, but decided to finish off the last ten feet anyway.

When I woke up the next morning I could barely turn my neck, and by the middle of the day my right shoulder and neck muscles were going into spasm constantly. I was at a conference, and when I got in the taxi to take me to the airport later in the afternoon, my neck seized up every time the taxi driver sped up, because the simple acceleration of the car made my neck fire in a similar way to the exercise that caused me to get hurt. I stabilized my neck and shoulders as best as I could and took a few days off from working out. Thankfully I was back to normal within about a week and a half, but it goes to show that a small twinge can have larger issues associated with it.

Commit to Consistency, but Vary Your Routine – It's important to do physical activity on a regular basis, but it doesn't matter so much what the activity is. So you may as well choose activities and workouts that you enjoy. If you do the same thing over and over, you may get bored with your exercise routine. So plan changes to your routine, whether you change an exercise or two or you completely shift your mode of exercising, such as transitioning from tennis to basketball or learning a new type of dance. Variety not only helps make consistency fun, it's also good for the brain. Learning new exercises and variations increases the neurological connections between your brain and body, which may increase cognitive function – meaning, you get smarter.

Get FITTE (pronounced "fit") – These are five basic variables of exercise. You can progress any of them to create a new stimulus for the body:

- Frequency – How often do you perform the activity each week or month?

- Intensity – How hard are you pushing yourself with the activity? How fast are you trying to move or how much resistance are you moving against?

- Time – How long are you performing the activity for?

- Type – Try a new type of activity or exercise.

- Enjoyment – Are you still enjoying the activity? We tend to stick with activities that we like, so make sure you're having fun! If you hate running, don't run. But try to figure out what causes the hate and if you can fix that. For example, if running hurts, see a specialist, physical therapist or trainer qualified in movement correction or gait analysis.

Get Uncomfortable – Doing a new activity, learning a new skill, working your legs instead of your arms for a change or trying to lift weights with each side of your body separately (unilateral) for the first time will all make you feel uncomfortable, because your body and brain are learning. Just like so many other parts of your health or fitness journey feel uncomfortable, this is no different. Feeling uncomfortable, however, is not about physical pain that indicates injury – it's about new sensations that indicate you're leaving your comfort zone, which is how you achieve new results!

Don't Get Hurt, Get a Coach – If you're new to exercise, get expert guidance from a trainer, coach or instructor: For a physical activity to be good for you, it must not injure you. Just like the Hippocratic Oath, "First do no harm." I've seen too many weight loss attempts get derailed by overzealous clients who decide to push themselves to work out five times a week—when they were doing nothing three weeks ago. Or people who try to do complex exercises like kettlebell swings without knowing how to use the equipment. If you're serious about your health, fitness and weight change pursuits, I strongly recommend investing in a coach, instructor or trainer for at least a few sessions to learn the basics of healthy movement in the physical activity you've chosen.

Move Better, then Move More – If you've been injured before, go see a physical therapist or movement correction specialist certified in the Functional Movement Screen. That person can work with you to correct your asymmetries and movement compensation patterns, which usually involves a healthy dose of myofascial release, stretching, trunk stability training and movement preparation. Doing that first will make your exercise routine much more beneficial in the long run.

Intensity Lets You Do More in Less Time – All trainers learn that when exercise intensity increases, duration should decrease. Jogging vs. sprinting is a good example. Jogging is a lower-intensity activity, so you can do it much longer. Try sprinting for half an hour—it's not going to happen! Usually we sprint for 15, 20, even 30 seconds, but much beyond that we're spent and need to slow down or stop and recover. After recovery, we can sprint again—and repeat. This is the essence of interval training. Remember this idea next time you think 20 minutes isn't enough time to get in a workout. A pair of sneakers and your body weight is all you need, and a five- to seven-minute warm-up leaves you with plenty of time for intense activity. Just remember that form and safety is most important.

Create a Balanced Workout – A balanced workout contains both push and pull exercises and both upper- and lower-body exercises. Because life happens in three dimensions, make sure your workouts do too. Multi-planar workouts include not only front-to-back exercises, but also side-to-side and rotational movements. Get more bang for your physical activity buck with exercises that move more than one joint at a time, like lat-pulldowns, pullups or rows instead of biceps curls. More joints involved means more muscles activated, which means more calories burned and more muscular lean mass primed to burn even more calories.

Training for a Particular Goal – If you're training for a particular goal, use the principle of specificity: train with activities similar to what you'll be doing in your event. For example, do some longer runs if you're preparing for a marathon, which requires significant levels of endurance, whereas a mixture of mid-range running and sprints will prepare you better for a soccer or basketball game, which requires a combination of power and endurance. Imagine what your body will be asked to do during your event and then train for it. At the same time, remember that trunk stability and coordination are important for performing your best and preventing injury during any activity, so keep a variety of exercises in your rotation. Focus on the goal, but cross-train to supplement and support.

Cardio Doesn't Have to Be Boring – Interval training is a great substitute for steady cardio, and you can do it with anything—from your favorite cardio machine such as the elliptical, treadmill or bike to bodyweight exercises or even battle ropes – those big tug-of-war ropes – and kettlebells. Just go for brief bouts of intense activity followed by a recovery period. For example, you could do 30 seconds of kettlebell swings followed by 30 seconds of rest and then repeat for 10 to 15 bouts, which would be 10 to 15 minutes total. See the *Advanced Cardiorespiratory Training: Intervals* section earlier in the chapter for more details.

Everyone Needs Resistance Training – Whether you are looking to lose weight, gain weight, increase strength, maintain your bone strength or prevent osteoporosis, moving your body against resistance is one of the most important parts of the equation. Feel free to use your bodyweight via squats, Pilates, yoga, dancing or lifting around the house, a partner via martial arts or wrestling, dumbbells, cables, kettlebells, exercise machines or soup cans and water jugs!

Do More in Less Time – Pair your exercises to work out more efficiently. During resistance workouts, I recommend doing pairs of push/pull or lower/upper body exercises. For example, you could pair squats with pushups. After using your lower body to do a set of squats you can immediately go into a set of pushups with your upper body, since the two exercises work different muscle groups. While you're working your upper body with the pushups, your lower body is recovering from the squats. And vice versa. Add on 30 to 60 seconds of rest after each pair of exercises.

Speed Isn't Just for Athletes – While you or your grandmother may not be aiming to win the Olympic 400-meter competition, you both need some form of speed and power – because you both still need to react quickly to your surroundings and environment at times. Kids and dogs run in front of us, we slip and trip, and people bump into us. We need to be able to react quickly to catch ourselves and avoid getting injured. One of the biggest factors in early death in people over 65 years of age is hip fracture as a result of a fall.

Your Brain is Boss – Our muscles aren't the brightest things in the world. Muscles only know how to do two things: contract and relax. So how are you able to miraculously coordinate the muscles in your body to do complex movements like walking, playing sports or even getting out of bed in the morning? The brain!

Become aware of how you move to make sure the right muscles are doing the work for you – for example, picking heavy stuff up from the ground using mostly your leg and butt muscles by squatting. As you consciously repeat the new movements, you'll strengthen the connection between your brain and the correct muscles. If you continue dangerous movement patterns, like lifting things with your lower back muscles by bending over, you'll be strengthening the wrong connections. And that's what leads to pain or injury.

Learn to Stabilize the Trunk – Know how to engage the scapular stabilizers, abdominals and glutes. Your knees, lower back and shoulders will thank you. Check out the *Engage the Trunk (aka the Core)* section earlier for more details.

TIPS TO PREVENT INJURY AND MUSCLE IMBALANCES

You don't want an injury to keep you from consistent exercise. In my humble opinion, the most preventable causes of exercise-related injuries are chronic movement and muscle imbalances, usually due to unhealthy movement patterns repeated for years. Three common causes are:

- Poor posture sustained all day, every day
- Exercising with poor movement patterns
- Improper movement learned when avoiding (no longer existent) pain from an old injury

Here are some tips to help fight movement imbalances and reduce your risk of injury:

1. Perform self-myofascial release and stretching frequently, at least as often as you're physically active. You may need more if you sit or stand for long periods of time during the day, or you move the same way over and over for work.

2. Stretch or move every 30 to 60 minutes when seated at work. Focus on the hip flexor stretch, chest stretch, squats or the tabletop downward dog:

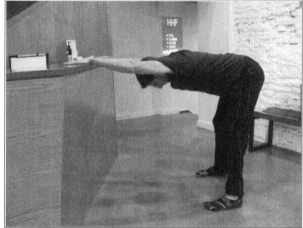

Tabletop Downward Dog

3. Arrange your workspace so that your hips and knees make 90-degree angles, your feet are firm-ly on the ground and you don't have to arch your neck or hunch forward to read or see a screen.

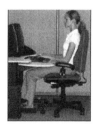

Photo Courtesy of Occupational Safety & Health Administration

4. Wear high heels only when you feel you really, really need to. Perform self-myofascial release on your feet and calves regularly if you do wear heels often.

5. Switch which side of your body you carry your bag on each day, or at least each week.

6. Try to minimize crossing your legs when you sit, or switch which leg you cross every so often. Same goes for shifting your weight to one leg when you stand.

7. Minimize sitting time, especially if you have to drive to work and then sit all day. Try to stand and walk or pace as much as you can, such as when on conference calls.

8. Strengthen your trunk stability by performing exercises that focus on keeping your mid-section steady – that's everywhere from just below the shoulders to just above the hips – as you move against resistance with your arms or legs.

9. Make sure your physical activity is balanced. For every "push" exercise there should be at least one "pull." If you sit a lot or hunch forward often, do two pulls for every push.

10. Listen to your body when you feel a chronic tightness or discomfort. It's usually a sign that something is out of whack and needs to be corrected. Take care of it before discomfort becomes pain, which eventually becomes injury!

11. See a qualified massage therapist or acupuncturist if some of your muscles are chronically tight. Sometimes we need a more precise instrument for myofascial release than a tennis ball or foam roller. That's where well-trained massage therapists' hands or acupuncturists' needles can release deep, built-up stresses in the body. Unless you want to go back to the massage therapist or acupuncturist regularly, however, you need to figure out the source of your chronic tightness and train to correct it.

HABIT 7: SIT LESS

RATIONALE

Sitting on your butt all day can kill you. Recent research has shown that being physically inactive for a large number of hours during the day – such as by sitting – could place you at risk for obesity and chronic disease even if you exercise. So if you have a desk job that keeps you seated six, eight or ten hours a day, being physically active is only half the battle. The other half is standing up.

Unfortunately, this appears to be a growing issue, especially in the U.S. *The New York Times* noted in 2011 that over the past fifty years, the percentage of U.S. jobs that require moderate levels of physical activity has plummeted from 50% to 20%. In other words, four out of five people barely move for a large portion of their day. And maybe you're then sitting for hours during a commute. And how about at home after work in front of the computer or TV? This inactivity can make you chronically tight in your hips and back. In addition, it leads to most of the conditions and diseases that physical activity fights against.

Why is sitting such a disaster? It's actually because of your legs. They contain your largest muscle groups, which mean they have the greatest potential to burn calories when used. Studies have looked at the muscle activity in peoples' legs when they were walking, standing and sitting. When you walk, your leg muscles fire with an active burst at each step. With standing, there's still a baseline level of muscle activity required for the legs to fight gravity and keep you up. When you sit, the activity of your legs flatlines, just like in an episode of a hospital drama. Get the defibrillator!

Less muscle activity = fewer calories burned throughout the day = greater risk for weight gain. Just standing can burn 20% to 30% more calories than sitting. So getting up regularly for a stretch, water or bathroom break can have a real impact. In fact, some people set up their desks so they can stand and work for a while – say, fifteen to twenty minutes standing each hour. Something is always better than nothing.

On the other hand, people with active jobs naturally burn more calories because they're on their feet and moving much of the day. However, this doesn't lead to better fitness unless they're working hard, such as in construction or sports, not just standing and walking. Improving fitness means planned physical activity (Habit #6) that pushes the body beyond what it's used to. So even those who have active jobs shouldn't forget the other important aspects of fitness such as cardiovascular, muscle and bone health.

Sitting is a natural part of your daily routine, but it shouldn't be the only thing you do all day. To quote Bob Marley: "get up, stand up!"

ASSESSMENT

Using the Physical Activity Tracker, simply count the number of hours you're seated every day for a week. Then add up your total hours spent sitting and divide by seven, the number of days in a week. The number you get will be your baseline average daily sitting time.

RECOMMENDATION

Aim to decrease your sitting time by one hour per day from your baseline daily average. You can stand, walk, exercise, hop in a circle, anything you want to do for that hour except sit or lie down. Of course, there are tips coming up on what to do.

EASY EIGHT HABIT #7 STRATEGIES

IF YOU MUST SIT...

Whether we like it or not, some jobs require sitting for extended periods of time. If you're in this situation, take a few steps to make sure sitting takes as little of a toll on your body as possible:

- Pay attention to your posture when sitting...get "tall" in your seat and engage your abs to stay tall. Imagine a string is pulling the crown of your head up to the ceiling.
- Get a memory foam or inflatable lumbar support. The support will

help, but don't use it to relax into poor posture.

- Engage your butt muscles to rock forward and back and side-to-side in your seat every few minutes, to get blood flowing and reduce stiffness in your lower body.

- You can always stretch your upper body when seated. With good posture, slowly turn your head and look to the left, to the right, up and then down. Always come back to center before moving to the next direction, rather than making circles, to avoid straining your neck.

- Do chin tucks to relieve pressure on your upper neck. Sit tall and lightly move your head back and chin down. It'll look like you're making a small double chin, and you'll probably feel a small stretch in the back of your neck. Perform ten times.

REPLACE SITTING WITH…?

So if I'm going to ask you to sit less, I should at least give you some ideas for what you can do instead, right? If you're not sitting, then you're either sleeping, standing or moving. Below you will find a bunch of ideas to replace your sitting time, depending on where you are during the day. If you can create just three opportunities per day to add some unplanned activity, you can lose up to three extra pounds per year, hassle-free.

Get Up at Work

- Lunge, skip or power walk to a co-worker's cubicle. Find an excuse to get out of the chair!

- Create a workstation that allows you to stand for part of the day. Use boxes, tables or chairs…get creative. I used to put my chair on my desk and then place my laptop on the chair…my computer was then at the right height for me to type while standing up.

- Stretch your arms and legs every time you get up from your chair. Think slow arm circles, self-hugs, stretching your chest in the doorway, calf pumps, downward dog with your hands on the desk, standing quad stretches, etc.

- Stand and move as much as possible while at work. You can stand during meetings, have "walk-meetings," or stand when on the phone.

- Drink more water at work so you need to get up and go to the bathroom more often. Double benefit: hydration and activity!

- Make it a game: Do a squat, jumping jack or push-up every time a common event happens at work, such as before a meeting, every time your boss calls you or when your co-worker with allergies sneezes.

- Do a different bodyweight exercise for 30 seconds every 30 to 60 minutes, such as squats, lunges, pushups, planks, jogging in place, mountain climbers or jumping jacks! 30 seconds of pushups are hard.

Get Up When You're Out and About

- Take the stairs whenever you can at home and at work, even if it's just a few flights. Then get on the elevator for the rest of the trip.

- When riding the elevator, do calf raises if there are other people there, or squats if you're alone or with a friend.

- Help your friends or family next time they move to a new house or apartment.

- Take public transportation when possible, as it usually involves standing and walking.

- If you don't mind looking slightly odd, try balancing on one leg while waiting on line.

Get Up at Home

- Make it a game: Do a squat, jumping jack or push-up every time a common event happens: opening a door, moving from room to room or when you or your significant other says a code word you've chosen together.

- Play an active game like charades.

- Clean your house or apartment with some elbow grease.

- Get up and cook a healthy meal rather than ordering in or sitting at a restaurant.

- Make some home repairs or build something for your home.

- Take your dog for more walks.

- Relieve your landscaping service and do your own yard work – be active and save money.

DECREASE OR CHANGE YOUR "SCREEN TIME"

While it may be difficult to control how much time you sit while at work, you can definitely control how much time you spend seated during your free time. The National Weight Control Registry, a database that tracks and studies the habits of thousands of people who have maintained at least thirty pounds of weight loss, found that 62% of the participants watch less than ten hours of television, Hulu or Netflix per week. That's less than one and a half hours per day. Reducing your screen time can have a huge impact on your hours seated each day – so here are a few ways to do it:

- Go retro…get rid of the remote control and change the channel by getting up.

- Do bodyweight exercises during commercial breaks when watching TV: squats, push-ups, jumping jacks, jogging in place, etc. That can be five minutes or more of exercise every half hour of TV time.

- Disconnect the TV: You will do more active things when you're not tempted to sit for hours in front of the screen. Test it out: Put your cable on hold for one month and see what you end up doing to fill the time.

- Play active video games like Dance, Dance Revolution, Kinect or Wii Fit.

- Play games that involve coordination, speed and skill, like table tennis or air hockey.

- Go outside. Play catch, make up a game or just roll around in the grass.

- Play with your kids...or someone else's kids (ask for permission first!).

TRY A NEW, ACTIVE HOBBY

The best way to reduce your screen time is to find something active that you would prefer to do instead of sitting and watching TV. There are probably hobbies that you've thought about doing but haven't taken action on. Start that hobby tomorrow. Here are a few ideas:

- Garden! Start a fruit and vegetable patch or a flower bed.

- Get in the garage and tinker or build something.

- Go dancing with a friend or significant other.

- For the daredevils, start indoor rock climbing.

- Go hiking with friends or join a hiking group.

- Go biking with friends or family, or bike to work. Sitting is ok in this case because you're actually working your legs.

HABIT 8: WALK MORE

RATIONALE

Just as you burn more calories when you're standing instead of sitting, you can burn even more calories by walking. Whether you're walking to work, around the office, during lunch, in the parking lot of a store, while window shopping or at home, increasing the steps you take each day can add up to better health, a lower risk of disease, better metabolism and extra pounds lost. And the difference between sitting, standing and walking is huge. Walking burns about twice the number of calories as standing and three times as many as sitting! Walking is a great option to kick your unplanned physical activity up another notch, especially if you have to be seated most of the day at work.

The suggested daily step count for health benefits is 10,000 steps, which equals about five miles. Your initial assessment may not be at that number, but any step you can take (pun intended) in the right direction is significant. A mile approximately equals 2000 steps and 100 calories burned. So increasing your daily step count by even 1000 steps per day, which is 12 minutes or so of walking, can save you over five pounds of weight gain every year – or cause that amount of weight loss.

And you can always take it a step further (ok, enough with the puns). You can get a lot more done than just strolling when you take more steps. You can take the dog for an extra walk, run around playing with your kids or move more by cleaning up around the house – your roommates or significant other will thank you. There will be lots of other ideas to increase your unplanned physical activity in the strategies section below.

ASSESSMENT

While you could count how many steps you take during the day, that would be slightly boring…and completely nuts! Luckily, a pedometer can do the job for you. Many options are available, ranging anywhere in price from $6 to $99*. Track your steps for three, four or seven days. The longer you track, the better. Include at least one weekend day, as physical activity habits are often different on the weekend.

Then take an average of the daily counts to get your assessment number. For example, if you took 5000 steps one day, 8000 steps another day and 9000 steps the third, the average would be 5000 + 8000 + 9000 = 22000 divided by 3 days (22000 / 3) = 7333 steps per day.

Note on Pedometers: The lower end models are "spring-based," which means every time you take a step and shake the pedometer up and down, it adds one to the count. You could actually just shake it yourself and see the count go up. Accelerometer-based pedometers are more accurate, but slightly more expensive. Finally, more advanced movement and activity monitors such as the FitBit pedometer can track stairs climbed, distance traveled and even how well you sleep.

RECOMMENDATION

Based on your average number of steps taken per day, aim to increase your daily steps taken by 500 to 1000 steps, which is equal to six to 12 extra minutes of walking. You can add them in anywhere, anytime throughout the day. In fact, studies show that walking briskly for at least ten minutes, three times per day can bring extra health benefits beyond calories burned.

EASY EIGHT HABIT #8 STRATEGIES

FIND SIX TO TWELVE MINUTES A DAY

As I mentioned before, getting an extra 500 to 1000 steps per day requires six to twelve minutes. So write down and review your daily schedule. Look for points during the day where you can spare that amount of time for a walk. If you want some help with this, the *Simple Strategies* section in Chapter 8 takes you through different parts of your daily routine where you can make a change.

LOOK FOR AND CREATE "WALKABLE MOMENTS"

Sometimes we don't plan for a walk, but the walk comes to us. Focusing your mind on spontaneous walking opportunities, or "walkable moments," will help you spot them in your daily life and routine. Here are some examples:

- Walk the golf course rather than taking a cart.
- Park your car farther away from work, the store or your house.
- Walk after a meal to aid digestion.
- Get off the subway or bus a stop or two early and walk.
- Take your dog for more walks.
- If they are manageable, carry your groceries from the store to your car rather than using a cart.
- Walk to stores that are within half a mile, or more if you'd like, from your home.
- Get up for a drink of water at work every 30 to 60 minutes.
- When you have to go to the bathroom at work, don't walk to the nearest bathroom, go to the one that's a little farther away. Unless you really have to go.

- Stand or walk during meetings at work. If it's a conference call, mute the call and walk around while you listen.
- Walk around the platform while waiting for a train.
- Do yard work: mow the lawn, rake some leaves, etc.
- Make it a point to walk *somewhere* every day.
- Walk while on vacation: Go sightseeing on foot, join a walking tour, walk around museums or go hiking.

WALK & TALK

We're all pretty good multi-taskers – you can probably do something else while you're walking. In fact, being focused on another activity, like talking, may allow you to walk even farther than you thought possible. If you're a social person, get others involved with your walking routine at home, at work or when you're out with friends.

- Go for a walk or run with a friend or significant other after a meal or before going out for the evening.
- Start a walking club at work. Walk ten or fifteen minutes every day around the parking lot or the halls in the morning, during lunch or in the afternoon.
- Have "walk meetings" with colleagues. A fifteen-minute meeting can also be a one-mile walk around the office.
- If you call someone to catch up, walk around as you talk. You may get into the conversation better as well.
- Join or form a hiking club. You can find or create a Meetup group (www.meetup.com). Or just go hiking with a friend while the two of you catch up.

COMMIT TO A 5K WALK SIX MONTHS FROM TODAY

A 5K (kilometer) run/walk is 3.1 miles, which translates to about 6200 steps. If you choose to increase your daily walking by 1000 steps each month (because it takes about four weeks to create a new habit) for the next six months, then by the end of six months you'll be walking three miles …the length of a 5K. Sign up for a charity that you care about, like Race for the Cure, to increase your commitment. Or you can sign up with a friend, and then start walking with them!

WALK PREPARED

If you intend to significantly increase your walking over the next few months, such as by signing up for a 5K, get ready for the new, healthy demands on your body:

- Get a comfortable pair of shoes; look for a local running or athletic shop, qualified trainer, physical therapist or podiatrist for guidance.

- A long, brisk walk is exercise, so do at least a brief warm-up or slower period of walking before picking up the pace.

- Have a glass of water an hour or two before longer walks, and then have a few gulps of water every fifteen minutes of walking.

- Maintain proper posture while walking to keep your joints and body feeling great. Good posture means keeping your spine long: imagine a string is pulling the crown of your head up to the sky. It also means keeping your abdominals engaged: pretend someone is going to punch you in the stomach. Finally, it means moving with your hips, not your lower back. You can adjust your stride to find what feels best.

BUILD A ROUTINE, THEN VARY IT

The first step to walking more is finding ways to do it consistently, usually by building it into your schedule. But once it's a solid part of your routine, you can change different aspects of the walk to keep yourself motivated, entertained and looking forward to it. Here are some ideas:

- Change where your walk for different surroundings. Even just walking your usual path in reverse can lead to new sights.

- Change your walking partner. Try meeting or catching up with a different person during your walks at work every day. Or go for a walk with one specific friend or member of your family each day so you can have some alone time with them.

- Change how you walk. Have you ever tried walking sideways or backwards? Try doing small ten to fifteen second intervals of sideways or backwards walking every minute or two during your walk. Be careful if you've never done this before, if you're walking on a bumpy surface or if you're still working on your balance.

- Change how fast you walk. Try doing small, ten to fifteen second bursts of faster, brisk walking every minute or two during your walk. Maintain good posture and slow down if something hurts – then get it checked out.

CHAPTER 8

MAKING CHANGE EVEN EASIER: PLANNING, SUPPORT AND GUIDANCE

The hardest part in the process of achieving long-term health, fitness or weight improvements is following through on a change consistently until it becomes a habit. Research has shown that it takes anywhere from three to as many as eight weeks for a new, *consistently performed* action, such as drinking one less soda per day, eating one more serving of vegetables or taking an extra thousand steps, to become a habit. And as you develop a new habit, odds are you're replacing an existing, less-healthy habit that requires conscious effort to break. Once your new action becomes your new habit, though, it actually becomes much easier to sustain since you've been doing it for weeks. It's no longer work; it's just a part of your routine, something you don't even think about. And with this new, positive habit comes new, positive results.

Making changes is much like running up a hill. The first few steps up the hill, like the first few times you take action on your decision to change, probably feel fine, even inspiring. But somewhere up the hill your legs start to burn, your heart beats faster and you get fatigued. At this point you are probably wondering whether you should have even attempted this damn run to begin with. You look over your shoulder and see the downhill path to where you were and it looks tempting. All too often we succumb to that return trip to our old habits. We stop, turn around and walk back to where we started rather than putting in the effort to push forward. Now imagine looking at that hill again a week or year later…do you think you will be more or less motivated and empowered to run up that hill the second, third or fourth time around if you did not succeed previously? Less, most likely, and that's why setting yourself up for success is the most important factor in taking consistent action on the changes needed to reach your desired health, fitness or weight results.

Many of the previous chapters have discussed ways to maximize your chances for success, such as:

Exploring why you want to change – This keeps you focused on why you want to make it up the hill. Imagine that your spouse, true love or best friend was waiting for you, or worse yet, their life depended on you getting to a town over that hill. Wouldn't you have done *anything* and *everything* it physically took to run, jog, walk or crawl to get over that hill?

Making small changes – Why try to climb Mount Everest tomorrow if you've never run up a hill before? You want to climb hills and make changes that are large enough to have an impact on your results, but not so big that it takes all of your effort to just get halfway up. Getting up smaller hills in the beginning can empower you to tackle larger hills and mountains in the future.

Focusing on one change at a time – Trying to make five small changes at once is the same as trying to juggle five balls at once…or stacking five small hills on top of each other. It just becomes one big mountain, and results in the same issues as trying to make a change that's too big. Also, you tend to get better at what you practice. Tackling changes one by one will give you the time, focus and energy to practice a change until you become an expert at it. Once you're an expert, then it's a habit and you can move on to the next hill without fear of slipping back down.

Despite the best of intentions and focusing on small changes, having the right preparation and support systems in place can make the journey much smoother and easier. Though you can succeed without them, it will be much more demanding, both physically and mentally. Why not make your climb as manageable as possible? This chapter will help you do just that, by:

1. Creating a practical plan for being consistent with your Easy Eight Habit change.

2. Building a strong support network around you that provides motivation and accountability while your new, healthy actions develop into permanent habits.

PLANNING: SIZING UP THE HILL

John Wooden, one of the most inspirational and successful collegiate basketball coaches, once said, "Failing to prepare is preparing to fail." While it is possible to succeed without having a plan, it's a hell of a lot harder. And when it comes to plans, something is always better than nothing. Imagine trying to give a speech or start a business by the seat of your pants, without any notes or information on your target market. On the flipside, planning shouldn't promote procrastination or create rigid marching orders. Rather, it's a way to create structured flexibility.

Planning to improve eating or physical activity habits can be boiled down into two components: strategies and evaluations.

Strategies provide clarity, and are mental preparation for the process of "practice, practice, practice;" that way, taking consistent action will be easier when you start making a change. Strategies give you time to consider the opportunities and roadblocks you may find when taking action on your chosen Easy Eight Habit. You can brainstorm solutions to anticipated challenges before they occur. By running through different situations and scenarios, like "what if I have to work late?" or "what if I go out to eat with friends?", you are focusing your mind on what you need to do to succeed rather than leaving yourself undefended against the whims of what you might "feel like doing" in the heat of the moment.

Then, as you begin to take consistent action, evaluations provide an opportunity to measure your progress (how far am I up the hill?) as well as make improvements along the way. For example, you may have to adjust to an unforeseen obstacle, like a change in your work schedule, a string of "special occasions," or an unanticipated stop at a buffet. Learning from these unexpected events and making them part of your plan allows you to be better prepared for similar events in the future.

Evaluations also give you a record to look back on and see all of your accomplishments. We are all prone to bad days, so having a record of previous successes and problem-solving strategies staring back at you can go a long way in keeping you focused, motivated and accountable.

If you're ever in doubt as to whether a particular planning idea is actually useful, just ask yourself: "How will this strategy or evaluation help me take consistent action more easily, either now or in the future?" If you cannot think of a good reason quickly, it may be worth shifting your focus to another, more impactful idea.

SUPPORT SYSTEMS: CREATING REFUELING STATIONS ON THE HILL

Support systems provide additional motivation and accountability as a way for you to stick to your Easy Eight Habit changes. It's like setting up "refueling stations" along the hill to make sure you feel just as confident about your journey halfway up as you do when you're just starting.

Motivation and accountability are the essences of these refueling stations. They create the "I can…", "I will…" and "I am…" feelings that override any doubts you may have. There are two types of motivation and accountability: internal and external. Each can be an important source of inspiration, which improves your ability to get results and achieve your Whys. Here's a brief description of each:

Internal Motivation and Accountability: Motivation is the feeling that you *want* to and *need* to stick to your Easy Eight Habit change and take the steps needed to get there. You recognize any limitations you may have and take steps to work on them, such as hiring a trainer for guidance if you know you are new to exercising. Internal motivation is heavily driven by your Whys. Accountability, on the other hand, is a self-created drive and responsibility to make sure you are making the best decisions for *you*, taking consistent action toward achieving your desired changes and being willing to take responsibility for when you are not. You must be willing to accept when things are not going according to plan and adjust accordingly. A great quote from *One Minute Manager* by Ken Blanchard and Spencer Johnson sums it up well: "We are not just our behavior, we are the person managing our behavior."

External Motivation and Accountability: You can get a lot of motivation through encouragement from people who inspire you to reach your goals. It can either be a direct statement, like "You can do it, one more exercise" or "You've been eating so well the past few weeks," or a push towards accountability like knowing that your workout buddy is going to meet you at 6 AM or that you'll be weighing in with a weight loss partner every Wednesday morning. This is a popular way of making sure you make the best decisions for yourself, because it's often easier for people to focus on making others happy or sticking to appointments, rather than self-regulating their decisions. This is a good option for those who find internal accountability challenging in the beginning.

Ultimately, internal motivation and accountability are the foundation of lasting change, because people, places and situations may change, but you will always be around – and have to manage – yourself. Creating a support system is crucial to help you get through tough times, but ultimately a strong sense of your own abilities – also known as self-confidence – will be what keeps you motivated and believing you can achieve permanent changes, get results and reach your Whys no matter what the situation. Ultimately, no one else can do your pushups, or eat healthfully for you. They can only drive you to *choose* to do it yourself.

DEFINE YOUR PLANS AND SUPPORT SYSTEMS

As you read through the different techniques for building plans, motivation and accountability, start brainstorming and write down which ones will be the most effective for getting you to take consistent action on your chosen Easy Eight Habit – it might help to write something specific, like "having a workout buddy who I go to the gym with on Mondays, Wednesdays and Fridays will be a source of external motivation and accountability to help me fulfill my Easy

Eight Habit goal of increasing the number of times I work out from two to three times a week."

As in the example above, one technique, like having a gym buddy, can fulfill more than one motivation and accountability need. Having a gym buddy can provide both external motivation (to get to the gym to have a great workout with a friend) and external accountability (because if you don't show up, he's without an exercise partner). The same goes for working with a fitness or nutrition professional. A few of my clients have hired me as a trainer for external accountability…they know they would not make it to the gym on their own, so I (and probably the money they spent) become their source of accountability and drive.

After reading this chapter, aim to have at least one source of motivation and accountability from both internal and external sources. Feel free to use the grid below. Make sure you feel confident that your chosen sources of motivation and accountability are the right ones for *you*.

My Sources of Internal Motivation & Accountability	*My Sources of External Motivation & Accountability*

THE HILL: REVISITED

So where does motivation, accountability and planning fit into the grand picture? Let's get back to the story of running up the hill. The key to *results* and long-term change is consistency and perseverance. With planning we can figure out how we will get up the hill of change, while motivation and accountability provide us with those short-term "refueling stations" along the way to help us get to the top where our actions become a habit.

Getting up that first hill – your first Easy Eight Habit – will probably create some new physical and mental challenges for you, especially if this is the first time you've tried to get up a hill that size. By having these refueling stations available, you will become reinvigorated despite the challenges and continue on. Once you ascend your hill and see the view from the top, the feeling of accomplishment will be a huge boost and will make the next challenge seem all that much easier. Imagine getting ready to run up your fourth hill having already successfully climbed three others.

And of course, now you get to enjoy the downhill ride on the other side of the hill! That downhill ride is when your new healthy action or step becomes a habit. Habits are sustained much more easily than a new action. So let's take a look at a few ways you can create plans and support systems to keep you focused and fueled on the climb to transform your planned *actions* into successful, positive, permanent *habits* that will ultimately create *results*.

PART 1: PLANNING

Redefining Willpower: Strategies

As I mentioned earlier in the book, willpower is not about extreme amounts of self-control. It's about having a straightforward plan, and motivating reasons (your Whys) to stick with it. Between your own personal experiences and reading the Easy Habit Strategies section of your chosen Easy Eight Habit, you're apt to have a lot of ideas on what you *could* change to successfully accomplish that new habit. The strategies you create to execute those ideas become your straightforward plan to turn actions into habits into results. Ultimately, you're defining what you are going to do and how you are going to do it, and making those steps as simple and easy as possible.

We are creatures of habit, so the best changes are the ones that fit into existing routines. Our strategies need to focus on doing just that: making the change as barely noticeable as possible to our inner frog – the one who hates boiling water. From working with my clients, I notice that most people's lives are divided into four routines:

- At home

- At work

- On the weekend

- Away from home/Traveling

Our days and weeks can vary from these routines, of course, so we need a little bit of structure and a little bit of adaptability. Creating a strategy to make your Easy Eight Habit part of each of your basic routines gives you a designated daily or weekly time to take action consistently. Planning via your established routines also gives you a chance to use your decision-making and problem-solving skills (practice, practice, practice!) for making healthy choices, because you have at least four options to accomplish your target action each day or week.

There's a template in the Appendix for filling out what strategies you'll use to change your existing routines. You are more than welcome to have more than one strategy per routine, and there's extra space to add in other routines that may not be covered by the four I listed above.

Once you've created strategies for your different routines, you need to figure out the best way to accomplish that strategy. In military terms, it's about defining the tactics you need to perform, or specific actions you can take, to achieve your strategy. Here's a basic example:

- *Habit:* Reducing indulgence frequency

- *Strategy:* "When I go out with friends on the weekend, I will have two fewer drinks – I usually have 4, now I'll have 2."

- *Tactic #1:* "Rather than having only beers when I go out drinking with friends, I will alternate one beer with one glass of water."

- *Tactic #2:* "After my second drink I will order club soda with a twist of lime so it looks like I have a drink."

Sometimes, you may need to keep many different variables in mind. For example, to increase your physical activity level an additional day per week (Habit #6), you may have to think about:

- Do I have to go to bed earlier to wake up earlier for a workout?

- Do I need to have exercise clothes with me during the day?

- Do I need to join a gym? Or purchase any new exercise equipment or clothes?

- Do I need to learn how to play a new sport or use a new piece of equipment?

It's not a bad idea to create a to-do list based on extra variables. If you currently run twice a week and want to start going to the gym to lift weights once a week after work, you could have a to-do list like this:

- Join the local gym.

- Buy workout clothes.

- Hire a trainer for three to five sessions to learn how to use the equipment.

- Put sneakers, shorts, t-shirt and toiletries in gym bag and put gym bag near front door or in my car before I go to bed.

- Make sure I have healthy leftovers handy, since when I get home after the workout I may be too tired or it may be too late to cook dinner from scratch.

- Go to bed by 11 PM so I get enough sleep to have energy left for my workout at the end of the day tomorrow.

Or if you wanted to add in a day of running in the morning before work:

- Buy running sneakers.

- Set alarm for 6 AM and move it away from the bed so I have to get up to turn it off.

- Go to bed by 11 PM so I get enough sleep to make sure I feel good for my run tomorrow morning.

- Sleep in my workout clothes (so I have absolutely no excuses!).

To find your best tactics, work backwards. With a strategy in mind, ask yourself: "What do I need to do to accomplish this strategy?" Write your answers down. Then for each answer you come up with, ask yourself, "How will I do that?" Write down your answers next to or below the previous answer. Keep on asking yourself "How will I do that?" and writing down your answers until you have a list of specific actions. Now you have your step-by-step list for achieving your strategy.

A common habit change that demonstrates this process is adding a mid-morning or mid-afternoon snack to your daily work routine that includes a fruit or vegetable (Habit #1 or #3). The questions that I typically ask for this change are as follows:

- What time will you have the snack?
- Will it be the same time every day or does it change? If it changes, when will you have it on those days?
- How much time do you have to eat the snack? Are you always on the run or can you stop for a few minutes?
- What are some snacks you would enjoy having (try to come up with 2 or 3)?
- How will you get the snack to work? Will you pick it up from a market on the way to work or will you prepare it at home?
- If you will pick it up from a market, which one and when?
- If you will prepare it at home, when would you prepare it? When would you buy the groceries to prepare it?

As you can see, even a small change such as adding a snack to your daily schedule requires coordinating many thoughts, efforts and actions. And since humans are able to process only about seven thoughts at a time, a small change can be plenty to keep you occupied. With time, repetition, practice and problem-solving, these efforts will become easier and eventually second nature. And that's when you can start focusing on another change.

WHEN CREATING STRATEGIES, LESS CAN BE MORE

A concept I originally came across while working with Core Performance, a corporate wellness program, is that the best strategies are the ones that can be done quickly, easily and without much added effort. Many of the Easy Eight Habits are based on this concept, and I want to discuss simple strategies in a bit more detail.

You may feel that going to the gym or starting a regimented set of eating habits is an overwhelming commitment at the moment, and that's fine. Simple strategies allow you to achieve your Easy Eight Habit within a couple of minutes during the day and build confidence for making future positive changes. The results of making these small changes repeatedly over time are similar to the effects of compound interest on saving money over time. While the fitness success stories and lottery winners are the ones that make the headlines, countless others (the vast majority, in fact) have amassed fortunes of health and wealth through small, consistent steps.

As the previous section discusses, existing activities and routines are the best place to start when you're looking to make positive changes to your eating or physical activity habits. Read through the lists below, and think about upgrading one or more of these aspects of your daily routine so it includes your chosen Easy Eight Habit. Credit goes to the Core Performance team for the foundation of these lists.

Daily Simple Strategy Opportunities

- Waking up
- Showering
- Brushing your teeth
- Eating breakfast
- Leaving the house
- Driving or commuting to work
- Arriving at work
- Setting up your desk
- Stocking your desk /drawers
- Transitioning between appointments or meetings

- Taking restroom breaks
- Eating lunch
- Packing up your desk
- Leaving work
- Driving or commuting home
- Entering the house
- Eating dinner
- Performing after dinner activities
- Brushing your teeth
- Going to bed

Routine-Based Simple Strategy Opportunities

Office activities
- Phone calls
- Meetings
- Desk work
- Breaks / lunch

Office "training equipment"
- Chair
- Doorway
- Desk
- Conference room
- Campus
- Stairs

Traveling
- At the airport
- On the plane
- Carrying luggage
- Post-flight
- Train? Bus?

Home activities
- Dog walking
- Washing the car
- Yard work / gardening
- Cleaning
- Playing with the kids

CHECK YOURSELF BEFORE YOU WRECK YOURSELF: EVALUATIONS

The vast majority of behavior, up to 90%, can be considered habitual. We get up, go to the bathroom, brush our teeth, shower, eat breakfast, etc. And that's just the first thirty to sixty minutes of our day! These habits have created desired results: We brush our teeth so we have good breath and don't get cavities. We shower to keep our skin and hair clean and healthy, while of course minimizing body odor. If we change our habits, the results will change. Imagine not showering for a week; what do you think would change? Would you get different results than the previous week when you showered regularly? In the end, habits create results and results don't lie.

Unfortunately, not all habits are so simple to track (like "don't shower = start to smell"). That's a pretty straightforward set of actions and consequences. Also, showering is a habit you are already performing (hopefully). For new or more complicated endeavors such as learning a new skill or making changes to your eating and physical activity habits, having a way to keep track of and review your *actions* is vital. By reviewing your daily actions and choices, you can find patterns and create accurate, constructive, non-judgmental feedback for yourself to help you accomplish your desired health, fitness and weight loss changes.

This section is focused on creating ways to track and monitor your progress on a particular Easy Eight Habit, and ultimately its results. As you would expect, the best evaluations are straightforward, easy to complete, and provide valuable feedback. The most important questions to ask yourself when developing your evaluation are *"What do I want to evaluate?"* and *"How often do I want to check it?"*

WHAT DO I WANT TO EVALUATE?

Choosing what to evaluate should be based on what is most important to you: your health, fitness or weight change desires, your Whys, your chosen Easy Eight Habit changes and any other activities that influence your ability to take consistent action on your Easy Eight Habit. For example, if you want to increase your workouts by one per week (Habit #6), you can plan, track and then evaluate your workouts throughout the week. From this information, you could make progressions and plan future workouts. Some other activities that can be worth tracking include:

How I Accomplished Today's Easy Eight Habit – If it worked for you today, odds are it'll work for you in the future. The more details you can provide, the better – who, what, where, why, when, how.

How I Intend to Accomplish Tomorrow's Easy Eight Habit – The best way to make sure something happens is to plan it out.

Tomorrow's Top Three To-Dos: It's easy to miss intended workouts and meals when you're inundated with unanticipated work. Fortunately, much of this work can usually be anticipated the night before when you take a couple minutes to reflect on it. If you plan and prioritize completing your most important tasks early in the day, it can free you up to do other important things: like eat vegetables and walk more.

Today's Achievements: All too often we only look at what we did wrong, without giving ourselves credit for our successes. We may get a great 30 minute run in before work, have a healthy bowl of oatmeal and berries for breakfast and a grilled chicken salad for lunch, but all we think about for the rest of the day is the two cookies we had in the afternoon. Then we deem ourselves a failure, so we have General Tso's chicken and fried rice for dinner and then ice cream for dessert since we've already screwed up.

If you can remind yourself daily about the great decisions you've made, then you'll be less likely to give up on yourself when you make a misstep in the future. Because in the end, you can see that it wasn't the two cookies that blew that healthy day. It was the *reaction* to the two cookies.

Problem Solving and Opportunities for Improvement: But let's say you did end up having General Tso's chicken, fried rice and ice cream that day. Giving yourself room to write down the situation, what led to it and how you can make improvements in similar, future situations gives you the opportunity to reflect, accept and change for the better. It's about progress, not perfection.

HOW OFTEN DO I WANT TO CHECK IT?

You want to check your Easy Eight Habits as often as you intend to make the changes. For example, let's say you want to track your daily fruit and vegetable intake to make sure you are getting one more per day (Habit #2)…in that case, track your actions daily. Even weekly changes, such as increasing your physical activity (Habit #6), may benefit from daily tracking because each day presents particular circumstances that do or do not allow you to get your workout in. The short-term impacts of these actions can also be tracked daily, such as energy or hunger levels. Ultimately, having more energy and not feeling starving all day are great indicators that your changes are likely effective, sustainable ones.

On the other hand, results that occur after your new action becomes a habit, such as changes in cholesterol, blood pressure, strength or weight should be evaluated less frequently, usually around once every four weeks. That's about how long it takes for a new action to become a habit. And habits are what produce results.

There's a weekly template for checking your progress in the Appendix. You should be able to fill out the evaluation in three to five minutes per day, and then you can read through your results for a few minutes at the end of each week. Feel free to adjust or tweak the template for your needs. There are also a few journals in the Appendix that you can use to track common short-term results and improvement opportunities like energy, hunger, stress or indulgences.

EXPECTING THE "UNEXPECTED"

In his book *The Success Principles*®, Jack Canfield (co-creator of the *Chicken Soup for the Soul*® series) provides a simple yet powerful equation that demonstrates the meaning of free will, or in health terms, "willpower." The equation is:

$$Event + Response = Outcome$$

As you go through your weight loss, health or fitness journey, you'll run into unexpected situations. In the equation, these are called "events." There will always be an upcoming vacation to deal with, visitors from out of town, holidays, late nights at work, unscheduled meetings, surprise events to attend, temper tantrums, etc. Although they seem like isolated incidents, we experience things like this all the time. For others, the events are even more pressing and consistent, such as working two jobs, being a single parent or taking care of a sick friend or relative. The key to getting the results you want and achieving your Whys is adjusting your *responses* to those events.

For example, imagine coming home from a long or stressful day at work. Many people's response to this event is to sit on the couch, zone out, eat a comfort food, go out for a drink with friends or generally do something to relax. This is the response part of the equation. For those who are looking to change their bodies by moving more or eating better, these responses are not in line with their Whys. As a result, they may feel guilty or discouraged when they choose a response that does not get them their desired outcome (becoming more active). This can start a vicious cycle of negative thoughts that leads to giving up and losing any initial progress they made.

But the beauty of this equation is that we can *change* our responses. Just like with any math equation, by changing our response, we can change the outcome. In the end, it all comes down to choice. We must *choose* to reject our usual responses that have gotten us our usual outcomes. We can perform better responses that will get us better outcomes!

At this point I'm sure you can think of at least a few ways to change your response to the event of returning from a long, stressful day: going home and cooking a tasty, healthy dinner, going out for a jog or working out at the gym, to name a few. Studies have shown that exercising releases endorphins – those "feel good" chemicals – so that once you finish your workout, you will feel much better than when you started. The key is *choosing* to start it, even if it means deciding to get up and move for just five minutes (which often becomes more once you're moving).

In summary, the best way to deal with unexpected events is to:

- Realize that not all unexpected events are truly unexpected.

- Create tactics to deal with expected "unexpected" events. Tactics can keep you motivated and guide your decisions during a moment of temptation or craving. The activity below can help you develop event-specific tactics.

- Always be improving. Create a way to learn from unexpected events that led to undesired responses and outcomes. There's more about dealing with challenges like this, or "roadblocks," in the next chapter.

Take action on these ideas right now – grab a piece of paper and make two columns, or use the space on the next page. Label one as "Event" and the other as "New Response." In the Event column, write down every expected or "unexpected" event you can think of that has impacted your ability to eat well or be physically active, either over the past month or from any previous time you've tried to make healthy changes and did not get your *desired* responses or outcomes. Some of these events may be difficult to acknowledge as barriers to living healthier, but write them anyway.

MY WILLPOWER TACTICS WORKSHEET	
Event	*New Response*

Here are some significant events that clients have included:

- Having a demanding job that makes them work long hours, through lunch, etc.
- Having to work two jobs to make ends meet.
- Having an inconsistent schedule.
- Having to take care of kids: multiple kids, single parent or both.

- Having to deal with an unsupportive significant other or relatives who may bring home unhealthy foods, entice you to make poor responses, etc.

Sometimes you cannot immediately change these aspects of your life. And that's the point. Some of these events are going to happen *no matter what*. The key will be the second step: how you *choose to respond* to those events.

Go back and start writing down "New Responses" to those events that will result in positive outcomes. It can be as simple as taking ten deep breaths when stressed instead of immediately reaching for junk food. Any response you write should be one that you can envision yourself planning for and doing to deal with the event. Having this list will go a long way in providing you with strategies for executing your Easy Eight Habits despite challenging situations. It will probably be easy to write down ideas for the first couple of minutes, but after a while it may become harder. The need for change can be very difficult to accept, but write down new responses anyway. The situations and exceptions to the routine that often trip people up and lead to lost momentum and motivation… you now have solutions for them. And amazingly, when you change some of your responses, not only do the outcomes change, but the events themselves may disappear or change for the better too!

Some potential solutions for common life situations:

- For kids, find day care or a relative to watch them for a couple hours a few times a week so you can exercise or cook.

- For a spouse, get them on board or ask them to respect your decision to change. Have a discussion about how their actions affect your efforts and make you feel.

- For an inconsistent schedule, write out your commitments and work schedule at the beginning of each week. Then plan out your exercise, cooking, meal times, etc. around your commitments. If conflicts occur, make choices according to your priorities. Sometimes it's just a matter of making a call or sending an email to reschedule one meeting that can make the difference.

- For not knowing how to eat or move better or needing more guidance, consider hiring a nutrition coach or fitness trainer. The key is to be clear about your budget, needs and goals. As someone who works in the field, I can tell you that passion (in your case, well-communicated Whys) can go a long way in convincing a fitness or nutrition professional to help you reach your goals. Rather than thinking of the money spent as a cost, try to see it as an investment in yourself and your long-term well-being:

  - A ten-pack of personal training sessions is a lot cheaper than a 10% co-pay on heart surgery or diabetes medication for the rest of your life.

  - How about all the money you spent in the past year on things that you rarely or never use? That money could be spent on improving your health, fitness or weight.

  - Consider using vacation money towards a health-based "staycation" this year for you and your family.

Remember the new definition of willpower: It's not about having to stare down a free cookie when you're hungry. It's about having a strategy to make sure that you either are not around the free cookies or have a healthier, satisfying snack on hand. It is possible to eat healthy just about anywhere, as long as you choose to put in the time, effort or focus to do so.

PART 2: CREATING SUPPORT SYSTEMS

THERE'S NO SUCH THING AS BAD PUBLICITY: SHARE YOUR VISION TO MOTIVATE YOURSELF...AND OTHERS!

Sharing your vision, goals, ideas and actions with others can be a huge motivating step in the right direction. Most people tend to go about it in one or both of these ways:

The small broadcast method – Speaking with close friends and family – those you trust. This can be a great way to open up some of your concerns or insecurities without feeling judged. Their ideas and feedback can be extremely valuable since they know you and your habits well, and have your best interests at heart. But they must be willing to be objective, non-judgmental and positive in the process. For your part, be aware if you have any tendencies to become defensive. Look to overcome those tendencies and integrate all of the useful feedback that you receive.

The large broadcast method – "Going public" and taking to the airwaves of community forums, like the local newspaper or community events, or social media like Facebook, Twitter or online threads, to get the word out that you are making positive changes to your eating and physical activity habits.

There are lots of other ways to broadcast your journey that are somewhere between these two styles:

- Post updates on your Facebook page or start a Facebook group related to your health, fitness or weight change journey. Or use any other social media outlet you prefer: Twitter, Pinterest, etc.

- Speak at a community event or write an article for the local newspaper about the changes you have made and what you've learned so far. If someone asks you for advice on their condition or situation, refer them to a qualified fitness or nutrition professional to minimize your liability risk.

- Speak with friends, family or colleagues who may be interested in making similar changes and create a small group focused on providing motivation and accountability. Set consistent meeting times.

- Create an in-person or online community forum or thread for questions and answers, a place for posting new ideas, providing feedback on ideas and actions taken, etc.

- Start a blog chronicling your journey – it will keep you focused and inspire others…and yourself!

- Motivate yourself by writing a post-dated check to a person or organization that you *do not* support – and send it to that person or organization if you do not achieve your health, fitness or weight change goal by the date on the check.

- Write and sign a pledge or contract that creates motivation. It can be a contract with your significant other, your children, yourself or your future self. You can combine this with the previous check idea.

- Commit to how you *will be* by setting a "weight loss" or "the new, healthy me" reveal party for the target date in the future when you intend to have achieved your desired health, fitness or weight changes. Make sure the time frame is realistic and in line with your Whys. Start inviting people to it now. Start planning all of the details of the party as if you are that new person: are you going to serve your guests healthy food? Is it potluck? What activities will be involved? Will it be an "active" party such as hiking, rafting or going for a walk?

In the end, the purpose of publicizing your changes is to create an environment, both internally and externally, that makes you feel supported, motivated and accountable. It's all about strengthening those personal commitments to yourself so you can make positive changes, achieve your Whys and live the life you want!

POSITIVITY AND NEGATIVITY ARE CONTAGIOUS: CHOOSE POSITIVITY

Think about the people you spend time with on a daily basis. Do they have the lifestyle you are striving to embrace? Are they making healthy decisions about their eating and physical activity habits? Do they generally have a positive mindset, not just about living healthier, but about life in general? The people you spend your time with can have a significant impact on your own thoughts and ability to make positive changes to your eating and physical activity habits.

This is because you tend to take on the emotions of the people around you. Being around depressed or angry people all the time will make you more sluggish or argumentative. And taking consistent action to improve your eating and physical activity habits requires energy. So if you're completely drained from being around negative people all day, do you think you'll be clamoring for your next workout, or looking for the nearest brownie? You only have so much positive energy to go around, so surround yourself with people that help increase your positive energy reserve, like supportive family, friends and co-workers, rather than drain it.

Take a piece of paper and title it: Creating my Positive People Environment, or use the space on the next page. Draw a line down the middle to split it into two columns. In the left column, write a big plus "+" sign and list all of the positive people you know in your life: The people who always seem to make you feel better when you are around them. The ones who inspire you to live better. The ones who are always looking to solve challenges rather than give up. The ones who usually succeed in their endeavors. The ones whom you wished you spent more time with.

Then in the right column, write a big minus "-" sign and list all of the negative people you know in your life – the ones who are not supportive of your decision to live healthier. They may be the people who always offer you less healthy foods, bring home junk food or make jokes or negative comments about your ability to take action on an Easy Eight Habit. They are also the folks who are always complaining, have something negative to say about everything and often have you feeling down, sad or frustrated after you are with them. You must be willing to list people based on how they make you feel, not on who they are – this includes your spouse, family and friends. That means you may have someone you care about end up in the minus column, and that's OK. We'll discuss how to deal with that soon.

CREATING MY POSITIVE PEOPLE ENVIRONMENT	
Positive: +	*Negative: -*

Take a look at the people on the "+" plus side of the paper and start spending more time with them, and if you can, doing some of the activities that they do. Start surrounding yourself with the people who inspire you to achieve the health, fitness or weight changes that you desire, or people who represent the final result that you want. A great way to become the type of person who is active four days a week and eats healthfully is to surround yourself with people who work out four days a week and eat healthfully, whether they are friends, family, health professionals or colleagues. You can ask them to mentor you, be a part of your support system, or just hang out for a day. The best way to learn is to speak with those who have already accomplished what you're striving for!

Now, take a look at the people on the "-" minus side. You can't always choose whom you spend your time with, but you can certainly change *how much* time you have to spend with them—the less the better. If you have a client that you can't stand and is always bringing you down, try to give that client to someone else. If you have co-workers who are always negative, minimize your time with them, sit far away from them at meetings and try to avoid working on team projects with them unless there are also more positive people on the team.

If you're close to your family but have one relative who's a constant downer or source of stress, tell that person how his actions or comments make you feel. Tell him that his actions and comments make you want to spend less time with him. That can be an eye opener and may motivate him to change, because he probably doesn't want to see less of you! Offer to work with your family member on turning those negative interactions into positive ones. If he can sense that you really do care about him, hopefully he'll be receptive to the offer to help. But if he refuses, then you've done all you can and must move on. You can't tell people how they should feel. In this case, the best option is to spend less time talking to him or being around him at family events.

If you do choose to spend time around negative people, you will have to learn how to deal with their negativity and let it run off of you as quickly as possible. Learn to become aware of their negativity and internally reject it; think of yourself as a negativity-free zone. It becomes easier to do this with practice, staying surrounded by positive people most of the time and, honestly, smiling often.

GET A LITTLE HELP FROM YOUR FRIENDS, FAMILY, PROFESSIONALS, COLLEAGUES...

You've got to be proactive and put in effort to create a support and guidance team, but it will pay tremendous dividends in the long run. These will be the people that you *know* you can turn to when you're feeling sluggish and negative, or are dealing with a significant roadblock. They are your "go-to" people for keeping you inspired, motivated and accountable for making positive changes to your eating habits and physical activity.

The best way to create this resource is to make a list of people, their role (nutrition or fitness professional, someone to call when you've had a crappy day, workout buddy, etc.) and their contact info. And of course, you need to ask them to be a part of your team!

MY SUPPORT & HEALTHCARE TEAM			
Name	*Role*	*Contact (Phone)*	*Contact (Email/Online)*

YOUR SUPPORT TEAM

Think about the people that can be there to motivate and inspire you when you need someone the most, regardless of whether they know a lot about nutrition, exercise or health. You can include the person you can call after you've had a long day and are looking for some stress release or inspiration to make healthy decisions. Or a friend who'd be willing to be your exercise buddy. Or a family member who can watch your child for an hour or two while you work out or shop for healthy foods.

These are the people who would forward you an interesting article about nutrition or health because they know you're trying to make positive changes.

Or they would be the ones to suggest a healthier restaurant or menu item when you're deciding where to go or what to eat. They also could be the people who inspire you through leading by example. Consider who of your friends, family or colleagues have successfully improved their health – they can be a valuable source of information and motivation.

YOUR HEALTHCARE TEAM

What better way to learn how to improve your health, fitness and weight than creating a list of professionals in the field that you know you can turn to for guidance and support? First, take stock of your existing professional relationships: your doctor(s), dietitian or nutritionist, chiropractor, personal trainer, coaches, etc. If you're dealing with any psychological concerns, including depression, a therapist would be a valuable member of your team.

Then, think about anyone in your network of family, friends, colleagues, etc. that has experience in the field you're looking to learn more about – nutrition, fitness, etc. Reach out to them to ask how they'd be willing to support you in your endeavors, such as by answering a few questions, discussing why you want to change or brainstorming ideas to put one of the Easy Eight Habits into practice.

MENTORING AND COACHING

Another valuable relationship you can establish is with a mentor or coach. This will be a person with whom you meet regularly for a given period of time, such as once every two weeks for thirty minutes, either in person or via Skype. Some of the members of your healthcare team can double down as a coach, particularly a dietitian or personal trainer. Just make sure they understand the roles of a mentor or coach.

Mentors and coaches both help you figure out how to do something better through advice, knowledge and previous experiences. They can also help you recognize if you've gone off course. Both should be able to provide you with resources and insights that you may not already have. Or they can serve as sounding boards while you brainstorm strategies.

Regarding payment or compensation, mentoring tends to be a bit more informal. Usually it involves asking a friend, family member or respected colleague to spend a little time with you. You can, and should, offer something in return – think about alternative ways of paying it back or forward. Maybe you have knowledge or experience in a field that your nutrition or exercise mentor needs help with, like advertising, finances, accounting, law, repairs, etc. You can create a bartering system where everyone wins.

Coaching, on the other hand, involves more than just giving advice, and you will probably hire a coach just as you would any other professional. Coaches act like navigators in your car of life. You're the driver since you know what works best for you, but coaches can provide guidance and ideas to get you to your destination faster or more safely. Coaches should have a background in behavior change and motivational interviewing. There are a number of resources to help you find coaches, such as WellCoaches, CoachU and MyBodyTutor.com. The key to finding a good coach is to speak with them about your goals, Whys and current habits and see how you feel while talking to them. If you feel that they "get you" and your situation, then they could be the right coach for you. On the other hand, if you feel they're not *listening* and are instead providing rigid responses that aren't tailored to you, then try looking elsewhere. A brief ten- to fifteen-minute conversation can tell you a lot about a potential coach.

Here are a few more pieces of advice for developing a successful mentoring or coaching relationship:

Know why you want to establish the relationship – Before you ask someone to mentor or coach you, know exactly how someone can help you – and tell them. Do you want them to give feedback on your eating habits and food records? Do you want them to review your exercise routine? Do you want them to be a source of new ideas? Also, the more you know about your own strengths and limitations, the better use you can make of your mentor or coach's time and abilities.

Be sensitive to the value of someone's time, including your own – Whether it's a professional or a friend, keep in mind that time is the most precious commodity for everyone. You may have to pay or compensate someone for professional, attentive services. You can pitch some bartering ideas, but try not to feel offended if someone prefers cash instead. At least you made the offer! On the flipside, remember your time, money and services are valuable as well. If you feel that your coach or mentor isn't valuing your time, tell them that and why you feel that way. If that does not get them back on track, then it may be worth finding another mentor or coach.

Be proactive in the relationship – Coaches and mentors can best help you if you want to help yourself. Coaching or mentoring clients who don't want to take the time and put in the effort to make changes is like trying to get a kid to leave Disney World. They may leave, but they'll go kicking and screaming. The more you know about yourself and how another person can help you, the sooner they can start making a difference in your journey. Remember, unless they are a friend or family member, they probably have no idea who you are and what your lifestyle is like when you first meet.

Act on the advice you get, and give your own feedback – A good coaching or mentoring session should end with a few ideas for progress that you can act on right away. The best thing you can do for everyone between then and the next session is simply to take action on those ideas and see how it goes. Did some things work? Did others not go according to plan? Did you get stuck somewhere? The more feedback you can give your mentor or coach, the better you two can handle any sticking points that come up. Coaching and mentoring is a dialogue, not a monologue.

MASTERMINDING: LEARNING AND SUPPORTING WITH OTHERS

In his landmark book about success, *Think and Grow Rich*, Napoleon Hill suggests creating a small network of people that can all turn to each other for advice and growth opportunities. He calls this a "Mastermind" group – a team of equals embarking on paths to improved health, fitness and weight change.

You can get a lot of insight from working with people from different backgrounds or with slightly different goals. For example, if you have a few friends or family members who are trying to lose weight, create a Mastermind group with them. But if you also have other friends who are trying to gain weight, add them into the mix as well. While they may have different goals from the rest of the group, they'll be dealing with making changes to the same elements in their lives, like eating the right foods consistently, performing the right kinds of physical activity regularly, overcoming challenges and looking for sources of motivation. Those that seem the most different may have much more in common than you think. And at the very least it gives everyone in the group a little more perspective in life.

Once you've formed your Mastermind group, usually between four to eight people, establish a regular meeting time and location. You might all get together twice a week, once every two weeks or once a month. Try organizing your Mastermind sessions in a format that gives everyone a chance to speak and receive feedback from the group. Here's an example:

1. Introductions and mingling.

2. Going around the circle, each person mentions recent successes and challenges while the other members in the group take notes on that person.

3. Celebrate both significant milestones and small wins. Simple acts of celebration can go a long way: a rousing round of applause or high-fives from the group.

4. The group then brainstorms on solutions for that person's challenges before moving to the next person. Make sure everyone feels _involved_ and _heard_.

5. Try using some of the publicizing and pledging techniques from earlier in the chapter within this group format.

6. The group could have pairs "buddy up" and become a part of each other's Support Team. Now everyone has someone to turn to independently of the group in case they are having a difficult time between Mastermind meetings.

COMMUNITY GROUPS: ANOTHER MASTERMINDING OPTION

In my opinion, people succeed with Weight Watchers® because of the community and social aspect, such as the weekly weigh-ins. Members know they will be weighed weekly, so there's a source of accountability. If they weigh less than that week, then everyone cheers and high-fives…it's great motivation! But when someone doesn't lose weight, or gains weight, you don't hear put-downs. The Weight Watchers team goes into problem-solving mode and asks the member how they felt that week, what decisions they made, etc. They brainstorm solutions for the following week together. And many members of the Weight Watchers team have lost weight themselves, so they feel an added camaraderie. That's the overall approach anyone in your positive people environment should be taking: supportive in both the good times and the not so good.

Other options for community groups include the local YMCA or gym, Overeaters Anonymous, local weight loss groups at community centers, religious organizations, local hospitals or online support groups, etc. Lots of options are out there – you just need to find them and join in.

GETTING THE MOST FROM YOUR SUPPORT SYSTEMS: ASK FOR GUIDANCE AND FEEDBACK

Once you've put in all the time and effort to create a support system, make sure you use it! Act on the guidance you get, and ask for help when you need it. Just like making positive changes to your eating and physical activity habits, the hardest part is not knowing what to do, but actually *doing* it. Answers and results come to those who go out and seek them.

Here are some common reasons for not fully using your support systems, and how to get around them:

Lack of Awareness – It never occurred to you that support systems are possible and useful. They are, and they are. Now you are aware.

Inconvenience for You – You may feel creating a support system and asking for help is inconvenient. If you feel this way, think about whether making positive changes to your eating and physical activity habits is really a priority for you. If it is, you'd want to set yourself up for success in every way possible, including having a support system.

Inconvenience for Others – You may feel you are inconveniencing the other person. How will you know until you ask?

Cost – You may feel it costs too much money. This means you choose to spend your money on other things – are those items more important to you than making changes to your eating or physical activity habits?

Fear of Rejection – You may fear being rejected by the people that you're asking for help. What's the worst that can happen? They can say "no." You're no worse off for having asked. If someone says "no," don't stress, just go to the next person. It's not your fault – it's probably because the person you asked is too busy or stressed out with their own lives. As long as you continue to ask, you *will* eventually get a "yes." I guarantee it (ask me).

Fear of Seeming Weak – Asking for help can feel uncomfortable if you think that it makes you seem weak or needy. Actually, it takes a strong person to ask for help – all of the best athletes and businesspeople have mentors or coaches.

Not Being Ready to Change – Fear of change or fear of failure can make you sabotage your own efforts, such as by not asking for help when you need it. If you're not asking for feedback because you think you know what you'll hear and you just don't want to hear it, you might be aiming for changes that are too big at this time. In that case, use your support system to brainstorm realistic, sustainable changes.

Avoiding Effort – Creating and maintaining a meaningful support system takes time, effort and practice. But eventually you'll have your team in place and they'll be a constant source of positivity for you. Isn't that worth a little upfront effort?

Here's one more tip – if people say yes to being a part of your healthcare, support or Mastermind team, you could have them sign a pledge stating what steps they'll take to help you reach your health, fitness or weight change desires – they could promise not to keep junk food in the house, choose better restaurants, watch the kids for an evening so you can go to the gym, etc.

By spending more time around your support system and healthcare team, and getting continual guidance from people who understand your point of view, you'll have a constant stream of new ideas tailored to your own goals. Then it is up to you to take action, practice, practice, practice and seek feedback.

ASK PERSONALIZED QUESTIONS TO GET PERSONALIZED FEEDBACK

Asking general questions – like "What are the best foods I can eat for X?" or "What exercises can I do for Y?" – gets you general information. On the other hand, asking questions specific to your own behavior will get you information you can really use. Here are some questions you can ask people who you trust will give you objective, non-judgmental, supportive feedback. Or you can even ask yourself:

"On a scale of 1-10, how would you rate my ability to do _____? What would it take to make it a 10?" Feel free to insert any concern into that blank, such as "eat healthy away from home," "consistently make it to the gym for my weekly workouts" or "cook a healthy dinner for myself."

"How do you see me limiting myself from achieving my (insert any Why, Easy Eight Habit, or strategy here)? What steps do you think I could take to get around this limitation?"

"Tell me where I could have been more _____ today/this week." You can ask about anything: general states of being (focused, energetic, positive) or specific actions such as "aware of healthy eating options around me," "able to plan my meals" or "focused on my physical activity."

ACCEPTING GUIDANCE AND FEEDBACK

The hardest part of getting feedback is accepting it and, if it's good, taking action on it. For many of us, our gut instinct is to get defensive, but the only way we can improve is to view the feedback as information to grow from. We must integrate feedback into our strategies and action plan. The best way to describe the ideal mindset for receiving guidance, advice and feedback is: *"Be teachable."*

If feedback about a particular action is positive, keep doing that action! If the feedback is consistently negative, or identifies a consistent challenge for you, view it as an improvement opportunity and adjust your course. Making adjustments will be discussed in the next chapter. Above all else, the last thing you want to do is cave in and quit based on some challenges or non-judgmental feedback that shows you need to make some serious changes.

Here are some thoughts to keep in mind when receiving feedback from others to make sure they'll want to continue helping you succeed:

- Be teachable by not just hearing their words but actually listening to their perspective and thoughts. Just as you would want to be listened to by a mentor or coach.

- Thank them for their time and honesty. Be grateful that they are willing to spend the time to support you in your health, fitness and weight change endeavors.

- Don't shoot the messenger.

- If the advice is good, take responsibility for the results of your actions and environment (don't just give up). Then take action to make improvements!

- Don't ignore the advice, even if you choose not to take it. Let them know why you ultimately chose not to integrate their feedback into your routine. And let them know you are very thankful for any future advice they continue to provide.

Finally, be aware of the source of the feedback. Supportive people may give you nutrition or exercise advice that they're not qualified to give. Better to double check the advice with a qualified member of your healthcare team. To sum it up: Ask. Take responsibility and action. Be grateful.

TAKING ACTION: SKIPPING STONES AND MAKING WAVES

When you start a new habit, it's like skipping a stone on a still pond. When the stone hits the water, it makes a change; not only does it create an impact, it also creates a series of waves that radiate away from the point of impact. These waves are similar to all of the other positive side effects of a single positive change, such as one of the Easy Eight Habits:

- Getting up to drink more water (Habit #4) will result in decreased sitting time and increase your daily step count (Habit #7 and #8).

- Increasing your meal frequency (Habit #1) or eating more fruits and vegetables (Habit #3) will likely make you less hungry at other meals so you'll eat less (Habit #2).

- Increasing your workout frequency (Habit #6) will probably increase your daily step count (Habit #7).

So by taking one positive action, you've set yourself up to take several other ones. And of course, stones usually don't skip just once. They create multiple impacts and multiple waves. Sometimes co-workers or family members notice your effort and get inspired to make their own changes. And then they ask you for guidance! Or as you start to make positive changes, you may meet other people who are interested in the same activities as you, like taking healthy cooking classes, dance lessons, hiking groups, gym buddies, etc. Before you know it, you're surrounded by a community of people looking to accomplish goals similar to yours…that can be motivating, and create accountability.

The key is to take action every day towards achieving your health, fitness or weight desires and Whys. With consistent action comes habits and with habits come results. As a bonus, consistent action often creates support, motivation and accountability, which is what keeps you fueled to get up the hill from action to habit. A formidable *positive* cycle. Keep this saying in mind:

I will strive to eat better and move more every day without guilt, restriction or injury.

And as you strive to maintain your habits and make improvements, it's all about feedback and adjustment.

The activities presented in this chapter have worked for different clients at different times based on their Whys, preferences and circumstances. If you're feeling a little overwhelmed, I have a simple, comprehensive planning & support tool to get you started at:

DeathoftheDiet.com/Chapter8Simplified

You can print, post and complete the form in about five minutes per month.

CHAPTER 9

THERE'S NO SUCH THING AS FAILURE, ONLY FEEDBACK

I'm going to admit it: I stretched the truth a little bit with the subtitle of my book. Starting a new habit is rarely easy. I should have named them "simple" habits, which is what they are: straightforward and actionable. That doesn't make them easy, though.

Here's another simple habit—saving for retirement. Put aside some money every paycheck, forego a few luxuries and in thirty or forty years, *poof*, we've created a nice little nest egg to enjoy in our golden years. Unfortunately, life doesn't always work out that way. We see that dress or watch in the store that we "need." Or we feel that we don't make enough to save while maintaining a reasonable lifestyle. Regardless of the reason, those who don't save today may be left wondering tomorrow why they can't retire at 60, 65, 70, or ever.

The problem is, our brains are hardwired to prefer fast, tangible results, particularly when stressed – so we often give in to immediate temptations. We also tend to overvalue an action's impact on the present (driving this new car makes me feel good and look cool) and undervalue its impact on the future (never mind the high monthly payments – I have twenty more years to save for retirement). Eventually, though, the future becomes the present; tomorrow becomes today.

And the same goes for adopting a healthier lifestyle of eating better or moving more. The payoff from eating a brownie when you're stressed or skipping exercise to get extra work done at the office is immediate: you feel less stressed or more productive. But is the short-term satisfaction worth the long-term impact? Consistently skipping your workout to get your assignments done early may land you a better job and more pay, but will you live long enough to enjoy it?

The plea of "eat better and move more for your long-term health" probably sounds like an overplayed tune. At the beginning of our first session, one of my clients told me that her goal was to lose weight and live more healthfully. When I asked her why and what losing weight would do for her, she said that she had a family history of diabetes and heart disease and she wanted to avoid the same fate as her relatives. Sounds like a pretty good rationale.

Later in the session she told me that she'd dropped about 25 pounds in preparation for a vacation she took a few months ago, but had since regained about eight of those pounds. The vacation was a close event with a tangible result (looking good in her bathing suit), so she put in the work to lose weight.

When I asked her about the recent weight regain, she said that when she went back to work after her vacation, she had nothing motivating her to stay physically active. I asked her about her initial desire to avoid heart disease or diabetes. She said, "Well, it is important…but I don't think I have to really worry about it at this point because I don't have the disease." So I asked her, "What do you think causes the disease?" Seems obvious, but it can be an eye-opener.

Unless you have a hot date, vacation, half marathon or some other pressing event happening every three months, odds are you will not prioritize getting in five workouts a week and skipping dessert six days a week.

And that's ok! Just like retirement savings are built up over a lifetime of small investments, so is a healthy lifestyle. In both cases, the best changes are the ones that don't make you feel like you're restricting or sacrificing. Because if you do feel that way, you will eventually rebel. Hopefully you're starting to see or feel results from one or more of the small, simple changes you've made to your habits.

Unfortunately, you can't set up an automatic savings plan for your health like David Bach recommends for your money in *The Automatic Millionaire*. You still need to feed yourself something at least three times a day, and no one else can do your pushups for you. And sticking to your Easy Eight Habit(s) every day, day in and day out for the rest of your life, is a significant task. So the goal of this final chapter is to prepare you for the times when things don't go according to plan.

READY, FIRE, AIM: BECAUSE NOT EVERYTHING GOES ACCORDING TO PLAN

You've already determined your Whys, chosen an Easy Eight Habit to focus on and planned how to take action on it. You're "ready." If you're already taking action on that plan, or are taking action as you create the plan, then you have "fired." But do you think your current plan is perfect? Do you think it will stay perfect forever? Or do you think it may still need some ironing out to get to your ultimate results? Now it's time to "aim."

Success, particularly when it comes to maintaining a healthy lifestyle, is a process. Life's a marathon, not a sprint. The same applies to taking action on the Easy Eight Habits and achieving your health, fitness and weight change desires. Imagine you've reached your goals and are living the life you want. Your work life, home life, relationships, spirituality and self-esteem are all where you want them to be.

How much longer would you like to continue feeling that way? Many people say, "forever." And that's a great answer. But that means you need to continue doing the things that got you there—which includes your eating and physical activity habits. So you must be willing to say goodbye to your old habits associated with your old self and embrace the new habits you've started—and will continue to maintain—forever.

Does that mean you'll do the same exact things every day for the rest of your life? No, you'll always be adjusting depending on your schedule, life events and other challenges that may come your way. But it's the mindset and strategies with which you approach these challenges that dictate your ultimate results.

There will always be circumstances you couldn't have anticipated, and they'll impact the plans you made to establish a new Easy Eight Habit. Sometimes you're able to come up with a good solution on the spot, and other times you're forced to make a less-than-ideal choice, like eating food that isn't the healthiest for you or skipping a workout.

Once that choice occurs, it has become an event. Here's Jack Canfield's equation again:

Event + Response = Outcome

You can't always control the events that happen in your life, but you can always control your response to them. And all events, whether good or bad, can only have one of two responses: a positive response or a negative one. And your *response* is what determines your *outcome*.

For example, you could have meetings pop up at the end of the day, or calls from friends asking you to go out in an hour…right when you were planning on working out! In that moment, let's say you choose to attend that meeting or go out with your friends and you miss your workout that day. You can view these events in one of two lights:

Negative Response: "Oh great, I blew it…this meeting (or social event) made me miss my workout so now I'm not going to burn enough calories today and I'm going to gain weight. This always happens: something comes up and I can't make my workout. Staying physically active consistently is never going to work; I may as well just give up now. Since I've decided not to work out anymore, I may as well have pizza tonight for dinner instead of the healthier meal I was planning."

Positive Response: "This unscheduled meeting (or social event) was a challenging situation, and now I see that my current strategies don't help me deal with it. This led to me missing my workout today, but now that I'm aware that situations like this can occur, I can plan for next time. If I'm going to an un-scheduled meeting, I'll see if I can work out after or fit the workout into another day that week. I'll also ask the manager who created the meeting to let me know what their planned meeting schedule is for the rest of the month, and find out what causes these unforeseen meetings to happen. Maybe we can figure out a way to avoid unplanned meetings in the future.

If the event is going out to dinner with my friends, I'll make sure that I make a healthy choice at dinner. Or I could tell my friends that I'll be a little late, because I'm going to workout first. Even a partial workout is better than none. I can also let my friends know what my workout schedule is so they can let me know about gatherings further in advance. That way I can reschedule my workout or they can even do the workout with me before we go out to din-ner!"

The event is the same, but the responses are completely different. That posi-tive response leads to a more productive mindset and a better outcome than the negative response, right? You may look at the positive response and think that it's completely unrealistic, but that is your *choice* to make.

A lot of things in your life that may seem like a foregone conclusion are actually flexible situations in which you have a choice. It's all about perception. Think about the movie "A Beautiful Mind," in which Russell Crowe plays the mathematician John Nash. Nash starts experiencing hallucinations – he sees people and experiences interactions that feel absolutely real to him. In actual-ity, the people he's talking to don't exist.

Some patterns you're used to may seem like concrete, unchangeable parts of life. When a pattern happens again and again, it can seem inevitable: a stress-ful day at work must lead to a pastry, or needing to take care of a child means no workout time for Mom or Dad.

In fact, you can always change your response. With commitment and ef-fort, it's possible to dictate your own response to any event…even debilitating hallucinations! At the end of the movie (warning, spoiler alert), Nash wins the

Nobel Prize. He turns and looks in the distance at three people who he now knows are hallucinations. He smiles and walks on with his family, now aware of what's real and what's not. While the hallucinations will always be in his life, Nash put in the effort to recognize them for what they are and chose to live the life he wanted despite their presence. In the end he was the one in control – not the hallucinations.

In the same way, you may never eliminate all of your cravings, but you can gain control over them. As you start to act on your Easy Eight Habit plans, you'll run into challenges. But eventually, the actions will become easier. And then they'll become habits. And then the habits – and the results from those habits – become a permanent part of who you are. You'll take it for granted that you're physically active three to four days a week, eat some fruits and veggies each day and rarely drink soda. You'll start to recognize the cravings that once controlled you as just that – impulses that you don't have to act on. You'll probably still have the occasional craving for a brownie after a long day of work, or feel like skipping your workout on a busy day, but with your strength and awareness, you'll finally have the power to choose to ignore those feelings.

To reach that point it takes lots of aiming: consistent action, positivity, persistence, receptiveness to feedback, and effective ways to cope with roadblocks and temptations. I can almost guarantee that you will come across new challenges and stresses between now and the rest of your life, some planned and some unplanned. People who are ultimately successful in maintaining their healthy lifestyle *no matter what* accept this fact:

You're always aiming. The process of positive lifestyle change is just a continuous, structured experiment of educated trial-and-error that you get better at over time. You can choose to develop your own personalized strategies for dealing with anything: a vacation, long day at the office or the chaos of the weekend.

The best long-term strategies are all about structured flexibility: enough structure so you know what steps to take when a challenge arises, but flexible enough for you to apply that strategy to different situations – such as eating at restaurants while at work, on vacation or over the weekend. Once you've internalized your healthy lifestyle, the feeling of success will last much longer than the initial exhilaration of reaching a target weight. You'll have it forever.

GIVE IT THE "OLD COLLEGE TRY" BY TRYING DIFFERENT STRATEGIES

When launching any new effort (writing a book comes to mind, for me), very few of us are perfect the first, second or third time around. It's a game of trial-and-error. Shawn Achor, author of *The Happiness Advantage*, calls it "falling up" – using mistakes and challenges as a motivating springboard to further progress. Finding the right solution takes time and perseverance. And that's why you need to give yourself at least three to four weeks to focus on turning your chosen Easy Eight action into a habit…just like we give babies time to learn how to walk.

It takes a baby about a year to learn how to travel on two feet. She's not born running around. First she must learn how to hold her head up, then roll over, then get on her hands and knees, then kneel and ultimately stand and take a step. But what happens on that first step? Usually she wobbles and falls over. Do we yell at her for being clumsy? No! We are super excited that she's trying, and encourage her to try again. Try, fall, repeat. Try, fall, repeat. And after enough practice, the baby will start to walk!

And for you, it's the same "baby steps." You've determined your Whys, chosen an Easy Eight Habit and started working on turning new actions into habits. Try an idea and see how it goes. Did you get the desired results? If so, keep it going! Or did you stumble a bit and need to adjust and try again? Every time you stumble, think of the baby and give yourself a pat on the back. Just as the baby learned that a particular movement didn't work for her, you now know a particular eating or physical activity idea isn't right for you at the moment. All ideas and strategies have merit, but they just need to be worked into your life at the right time. It's like buying that baby who just learned to walk a new car: good idea, about seventeen years too early.

Alternately, you can be cruising along, getting results with your improved eating and physical activity habits, and then you run into a roadblock. Roadblocks are external circumstances that force you to change your habits. Your commitment to achieving your desired health, fitness or weight changes, and your passion for your Whys, may be tested during these times. But roadblocks are a part of the natural course of events, and they do have an upside…they let you know you're on the right track! The key is to not feel defeated. Instead, figure out how to deal with or get around them.

Here's an example: Lewis and Clark blazed a path across the United States filled with many pitfalls and roadblocks—literally! Dense forests, canyons, huge mountains, unforgiving weather and lots of hostile situations. When they hit the first wide river, did they turn around and go home? Nope. How about when they saw the Rocky Mountains staring at them in the distance? Nope – and they didn't have an airplane. Reaching the other end of the country was their Why, and they got there, come hell, high water or both.

Roadblocks are anything that stands in the way of accomplishing or maintaining your Whys. They can be big or small, positive or negative, such as: unforeseen work deadlines, an unannounced meeting, the birth of a child, an injury, a stressful day at home or work, getting married, switching jobs, moving, losing your workout buddy, seeing slower results from your changes, losing motivation, etc. Sometimes you make the right decision in the moment of confronting a roadblock, and other times you may give in to a temptation or craving. In some cases you may feel lost and not know what the right decision is. When facing a roadblock, here are a few non-ideal responses:

- Get frustrated, blame the situation for your actions and give up on your entire journey.
- Wallow in self-pity, label yourself a failure, conclude that you don't deserve to reach your life goals and give up on your entire journey.
- Ignore the roadblock, particularly if it is (or will be) a recurring issue.

Running into a roadblock is not a sign of failure. They are actually necessary for improvement, and creating positive responses to them is an important step on the path to success. The first thing to do when you hit a roadblock is accept the situation and any feelings associated with it. Then do all you can to fix the problem in the moment. Afterwards, become solution-oriented and strategize ways to avoid or work around that roadblock in the future. Strategizing solutions to your healthy eating and activity roadblocks is like having spare tires – or permanent replacements – in the car to deal with any roadblock that causes a flat. Here's a great method for approaching and dealing with roadblocks:

1. Write down your roadblock, temptation or craving as soon as it happens. Be as specific about it as possible.

2. Pause for a moment and take a deep breath while thinking about the roadblock. How does it make you feel?

3. Write down any negative responses you may have made to the roadblock, such as giving into a temptation or craving, or moving away from one of your Whys, to get them "out of your system."

4. Focus on how much you value yourself and how much you have already done. Write down those accomplishments, too. You can review your Whys and the successes listed in your evaluations for a renewed sense of focus.

5. Think about how to improve and then move on! Be solution-oriented by brainstorming at least two strategies for getting around a roadblock. Use the Easy Eight Habit strategy sections or talk to some of your support and guidance crew.

6. Then take action on those strategies and see what happens! Receive feedback. Adjust. Receive feedback. Adjust.

TURNING NEGATIVE RESPONSES INTO POSITIVE ONES: ROADBLOCKS, FEEDBACK AND PATTERN RECOGNITION

My Road-block	How I Feel/ Felt	Negative Responses	Why I'm Awesome	Two Ways I Can Get Around the Roadblock

IF AT FIRST YOU DON'T SUCCEED... (AKA WHY THERE ARE EIGHT EASY HABITS)

"Goals begin behavior. Consequences maintain or change them." This quote from *One Minute Manager* by Ken Blanchard and Spencer Johnson perfectly represents the concepts of action, results, feedback and adjustment. When you take actions consistently, your body will reflect the results of those new habits. You must then be receptive to the feedback from those results, whether good or bad, by listening both internally and externally:

- Does a particular exercise cause pain? If so, make sure you can keep active without injuring yourself by asking or hiring a trainer to suggest a substitute exercise.

- Does eating a big meal cause you to feel sluggish? Think about whether that indulgence is worth it.

- Does having a big salad with some lean protein and whole grains give you lots of energy? Then keep doing it!

- Are people commenting that you are looking thinner, even if you didn't lose any weight? Muscle weighs more than fat but takes up less space. If your clothes fit better, that's a good sign!

Pay attention to patterns. When you experience a negative response and a negative outcome, it's actually a "feedback situation" – a chance to improve. If the same feedback situation comes up once or twice, it could be an unforeseen circumstance, and you can brainstorm ways to be ready for it. If it's occurring repeatedly, however, despite the fact that you're adjusting your strategies each time, you may need to focus on a different Easy Eight Habit.

Picking up on these subtle sources of feedback can mean the difference between focusing on feelings of success vs. frustration. After you've been taking consistent action on an Easy Eight Habit for a few weeks, stop and take a look at your progress. Read through your daily evaluations – what changes have stuck? What emotions have accompanied your progress? Ask yourself: "Do my actions match my goals and desires?" If so, keep going! Feel free to choose another Easy Eight Habit to work on if you want further results.

If you feel that your actions and habits haven't matched your desires, think about what needs to change. If you've given your chosen Easy Eight Habit the "old college try" for several weeks and haven't been able to convert it from an action to a habit, try another habit change – that's why there are eight! Based on your schedule, priorities and preferences, different habits can work for you at different times in your life. Be receptive to each of them based on the feedback you experience. If one change doesn't stick, another one probably will – here are some examples:

- Does your busy schedule keep you from getting an extra workout in? (Habit #6) Try sitting less or walking more during the workday. (Habit #7 or #8)

- Do you hate fruits and vegetables, and you tried a bunch more and still hate them? (Habit #3) It might be easier to reduce your meal sizes instead. (Habit #2)

- Do you consistently cut out one indulgence…only to replace it with a new one later in the week? (Habit #5) Consider adding a fruit or veggie snack to your daily routine. (Habit #3)

- Have you reduced your portion sizes, but now find yourself starving and tempted to eat junk food all day? (Habit #2) Eat more often instead, with a healthy snack such as a fruit or veggie when you feel most hungry. (Habit #1 and #3)

If you're not sure where to start, just drink more water. (Habit #4) Staying hydrated can have a ripple effect across your day, from increased energy to fewer cravings, which will make it easier to achieve other Easy Eight Habits.

Success is only a matter of time and practice when you believe that there is no such thing as failure, only feedback.

STILL STUCK? OTHER OPTIONS

If you've been working on the Easy Eight Habit changes for a while (at least three to six months) without getting any results, and you can't figure out what's causing the roadblock, here are a few things you can do:

Ask for Feedback

Start by asking yourself a few questions and answering them truthfully:

- Am I still motivated to achieve my Whys? Are my Whys what I want to accomplish or have other desires become more important to me?

- Am I really taking consistent action, or do I just tell myself that I am? Am I not being totally truthful about my actions and habits on my evaluations?

- Am I recognizing the results I do get? What results *am* I achieving with my current habits?

If your old habits were leading to weight gain, and now you're maintaining your weight, that's progress. Do you have more energy during the day with your current habits? That's progress. If questions like that don't reveal any progress you hadn't noticed before, and you still feel frustrated, feedback from other people could help. Often objective feedback from others can uncover solutions that had been hiding under our noses the entire time:

Get feedback from your support system – Consider asking a trusted friend, family member or colleague for some honest feedback about what may be limiting you. Maybe you don't realize that your workouts are much less focused than they used to be, or that you're indulging a bit more often than you used to. Be receptive to their feedback, thank them and then act on it!

Go to a professional for guidance – A dietitian, personal trainer or health coach will review your routines to see where there's room for improvement and changes. Sometimes it's all about getting an outside source of ideas to refocus and motivate you. Or the professional may push you to be more accountable for the results of your choices.

Get a professional feedback service – So far, I've only come across two forms of organized feedback aimed at improving health habits. One option is hiring a nutrition or fitness coach and meeting regularly to review the ideas in this book. Remember, knowing what's in this book is one thing; taking action on it is another! Coaches will help you convert knowledge into action. The other form of organized feedback is a coaching service called My Body Tutor (www.MyBodyTutor.com). The founder, Adam Gilbert, writes that his entire site is designed to help people "stay consistent" with their positive eating and physical activity changes. Having met him and seen his work firsthand, I'm a huge proponent of the service. If it's within your budget, I recommend it.

OTHER LIFESTYLE DECISIONS

Other lifestyle factors play a role in your ability to form more positive habits. Becoming aware of these factors is the first step to taking action on them. A few of the most notable examples are smoking, stress and sleep. You want to get these lifestyle habits "in your corner" to make your health, fitness or weight improvement journey as easy as possible.

Smoking – Most people who smoke know that they shouldn't, but choose to anyway for a number of reasons. They're aware of the serious damage that they are causing their body, the negative impact it has on their ability to be physically active – it destroys endurance – and the increased likelihood of heart disease and cancer.

Interestingly, smoking is associated with other negative lifestyle factors such as drinking, poor diet and low activity levels. Maybe some people feel that doing one unhealthy thing, like smoking, licenses them to choose a totally unhealthy lifestyle. Or they might feel that because they smoke, they are unhealthy – and then they give in to this negative perception of themselves.

Quitting smoking can be tough, because it's frequently used as a coping mechanism for stress, and if someone quits smoking they must find another way to deal with stress. Often it becomes food – that's why weight gain is common after quitting smoking. Other ways to deal with stress include exercise, meditation, or relaxing hobbies like cooking, playing an instrument, knitting, etc.

Overcome Chronic Stress – Single, intense bouts of stress, such as a one-time presentation or an exercise session, can push the body to improve. However, chronic stress can harm your body – it triggers hormonal and inflammatory responses that cause you to have unbalanced blood sugar, eat more, crave more unhealthy food and be more likely to gain fat. That's why reducing stress is beneficial beyond just "feeling relaxed." It can get you healthy and help you lose fat! Here are some ideas to help:

- Meditate.
- Pray.
- Take a yoga class.
- Do one of your favorite relaxing hobbies.
- Focus on doing less, but doing it better. Delegate more responsibilities or learn to say "No" to some requests. If you overbook yourself, you may feel too overwhelmed to make even a small change like an Easy Eight Habit.
- Practice breathing through your stomach by sitting up straight or lying on your back, closing your eyes, placing your hand on your stomach and using your breath to gently and slowly push your stomach into your hand ten times. This is called diaphragmatic breathing.

- Visualize your health, fitness or weight change desires and Whys for ten minutes.

- Plan your next day the night before and write down your to-do list.

- Prepare your meals and get your workout clothes ready the night before.

- Move more or eat better…that will naturally improve stress levels!

Sleep – Your body reacts to sleep deprivation a lot like it does to chronic stress. Studies show that you eat more, are more susceptible to cravings and less able to initiate change – for example, going to the gym an extra day per week – when you're sleep deprived. You may also have trouble kicking a caffeine addiction if you're always sleepy. Gradually increase your sleep to at least six hours – ideally seven to eight – per night. You could feel more fatigued at first, as your body starts to crave the sleep it has wanted for a long time. Once you refill your body's sleep reservoirs you'll find that your energy levels, focus, productivity and ability to make healthier decisions will improve.

RETHINK YOUR PRIORITIES

Grab a piece of paper and write down how many commitments you have. Include your job(s), family, volunteering, hobbies, etc. Next to each commitment, write down everything you need to do on a daily or weekly basis to fulfill your obligations to that element in your life. Then, add all of the activities and commitments you *want* to be doing, such as exercising more or preparing healthy meals. It can add up!

All of these commitments and their associated tasks can weigh on your mind, especially if they need to be done *every* day or week. They may become a serious drain on your ability to focus your efforts on other, possibly more important, activities like becoming more active and eating better.

For example, if you're constantly worrying about fulfilling your next commitment, rushing from work to childcare to household chores to your volunteer activity, then your mind is never free to consider a change. When you're stressing about your packed day, you're not thinking about what healthy meal you want to prepare for dinner, or what exercise you'll do that evening. Or, all that anxiety keeps you from focusing at work, so you're up past your bedtime finishing everything at night. As a result, you get less sleep than you wanted, which leads to increased stress and poor eating and physical activity decisions the next day.

All too often, an overload of commitments becomes a distraction that stays with us day after day, week after week, and we're always trying to catch up rather than progress forward. It becomes an underlying, subconscious source of chronic stress than can wreak havoc on us mentally and physically. As mentioned earlier, chronic stress can show up in your life in many ways: poor sleep (have you ever had trouble falling asleep at night with thoughts racing through your mind?), stress eating, or a constant feeling of fatigue that makes it harder to stay active. When everyday life is so overwhelming, you might be too exhausted to sort through your commitments and evaluate them. Emotional hoarding, if you will. While eating well and being active can help you become focused and more efficient, sometimes you need to break through the chronic stress first before you can take other positive steps in your life.

One of the best techniques I've come across to overcome these distractions is the four D's. Look through your current commitments and activities and choose one of the four D's for each of them:

PRIORITIZING MY HEALTH, FITNESS AND NUTRITION

My Commitments	Do	Delegate	Delay (when)	Dump

Do – Nike's slogan says it best: Just Do It. If you can, tie up any loose ends by finishing the commitment: whether it is catching up on emails, finishing a book or completing a project at home or work. Focus your energy on completing the task and then it will be done and out of your mind.

Delegate – If you can have someone else take care of the commitment or activity for you, then by all means delegate. The best managers – and this includes self-management – know how to delegate responsibility to those who are capable of accomplishing the activity. Delegating an activity may require an upfront investment of time to train someone else to do the activity properly, but once delegated, you'll be freed up to focus on what you want.

Do you have a friend, intern, colleague or child who can be responsible for some of your commitments? Delegation may seem like just dumping your work on others, but that's simply not true. If you're really worried about freeloading, the best thing to do is to speak with the person you want to delegate your activity to, tell them why you want to delegate it and ask how they feel about taking on the responsibility. Many people like having greater responsibility; it makes them feel accomplished and it helps them learn and grow as well. Odds are they will be happy to help!

For example, you can show your kids how to do the dishes, teach your significant other how to cook or show your assistant how to handle some additional paperwork so you can get a couple workouts in every week. You can even create a delegate list broken down into three sections: the activity, who to delegate it to and what you need to do to be sure you can completely delegate it. Does the person need training? Do you need to watch the first couple of times to make sure the activity is performed correctly? The goal should be that once you are done investing your time in training the person to perform the activity, you shouldn't have to worry about it ever again (or at least rarely…kids and assistants are allowed to get sick once in a while).

Delay – If you cannot Do it immediately and cannot Delegate the responsibility to someone else, then you may have to Dump the activity or commitment. However, if your gut or heart is screaming, "No, don't give that up, it's too important!" you can consider delaying it. There are two ways to delay:

Choose to delay an activity or commitment for a specified period of time, anywhere from a few weeks to a few months, and then re-address it. When you commit to delaying, that means you *will not* think about the activity again until that designated point in time. In other words, it will not take up space in your brain until either you are ready to Do it or the "Delay date" comes. When that time comes, reconsider the Do or Delegate options. If you still cannot Do or Delegate, then Dump it – because you've already delayed it once and still chose not to Do it.

Or, create a plan to complete the activity or commitment. If you cannot work on something right now but know that you will have the time very soon, create a specific plan on how, what and when you will complete this task, including a completion date. If you reach the date of completion and you've barely done anything on this activity or commitment, again odds are you should Dump it.

Dump – Dumping some commitments can be easy, but it can also be very hard, especially if we made a commitment to someone we care about. All too often we dump the commitments to ourselves, like eating healthfully and being active, for the commitments we make to others – and that's the problem. There comes a time when we must say "enough is enough" and let go of the unrealistic expectations we have of ourselves.

If you're dumping a significant commitment, the best thing to do is to be upfront and sincere about it. Dump commitments graciously. Acknowledge that you had made the commitment, but unfortunately due to changing priorities – you've decided to live a healthier life – you can no longer effectively fulfill the role you had initially committed to. It's much better to acknowledge that you're overextended than to stick around and do a lousy job.

By stepping away from a commitment you cannot fulfill, you're freeing that manager, friend or family member to find someone who can help them as much as possible. Everyone wins. Do your best to help the person transition the activities to someone else if you can, but in the end you need it off *your* plate. A person who really cares about you and your well-being will understand your change in priorities.

CHECK YOUR HORMONES AND LAB VALUES

Hormone imbalances and nutrient deficiencies can really hamper your efforts to be active and eat better, particularly a condition called hypothyroidism, or underactive thyroid, which slows your metabolism and often results in fatigue. Dr. Daniel Amen, a clinical psychologist, wrote a book called *Change Your Brain, Change Your Body* that has a list of hormones and conditions that can impact your metabolism, energy levels and focus. You can request to have any of them tested at your next yearly physical: complete blood count, metabolic panel, vitamin B12, vitamin D, folic acid, blood lipids, fasting glucose, thyroid, testosterone, estrogen, progesterone and fatty acid profiles.

Having a clean bill of health can give you the peace of mind of knowing that you don't have any underlying conditions making positive change more difficult. And if you do have a condition, you're now aware that it exists so you can do something about it! Remember, it's all about making change as easy as possible, and having your body functioning properly will make it more adaptable to change.

CHECK FOR FOOD ALLERGIES/SENSITIVITIES

Being allergic, intolerant, or sensitive to certain foods can cause very uncomfortable reactions, including bloating, gas, hives, diarrhea, headaches, migraines, fibromyalgia, IBS and even trouble breathing. You usually know if you're significantly allergic to a food, such as nuts, milk, soy, wheat, or shellfish. Other times you're just intolerant to the food, which is the case with people who are lactose intolerant and have trouble digesting dairy products. A number of allergy and food intolerance tests are available, so discuss this with your doctor if you believe you may be allergic or intolerant to a particular food.

However, you can also become "sensitive" to foods without a classic allergic reaction. This often results from having too much of it over a long period of time, such as multiple times per day, every day, for years. For example, a lot of people these days are concerned about gluten, which is most commonly found in wheat. Most people are not allergic to gluten, but some may have developed sensitivities to it because they eat wheat cereal for breakfast, wheat bread with lunch and whole wheat pasta for dinner.

When you're exposed to a food that frequently, your immune system could begin to react to the food with the symptoms mentioned above. Unfortunately, this immune response cannot be measured by traditional allergy tests. These food sensitivities can be difficult to address because the symptoms arise for so many reasons: different foods consumed in different amounts resulting in inflammation from different sources within the body.

The only test that I know of that measures food sensitivities is the Mediator Release Test (MRT), developed by Oxford Biomedical Technologies. It's a blood test that measures your sensitivity to 150 different foods and additives. In addition, you receive a lifestyle-based program tailored to the results of your test called Lifestyle Eating and Performance Therapy (LEAP therapy). You can find certified LEAP therapists across the country. I've included a link to the MRT and LEAP websites in the Appendix.

DEALING WITH "GAME CHANGERS"

Ever try to drive a car on a flat tire? It'll go for a while, but you're eventually going to have to take it into the shop to get it checked out. It would be better to address the flat tire sooner, while you're still going strong, rather than later—when you're frustrated and broken down on the side of the highway.

Trying to make positive lifestyle changes and get results, while ignoring some other significant change in your life, is just like driving with a flat tire. Game changers, whether good or bad, are times in life when there's a radical shift in schedule or demands – and these often have a significant impact on your physical activity or eating habits. Some are planned while others are not. The better you can prepare and plan for one, the easier the transition will be, but sometimes it becomes another game of educated trial-and-error.

Below is a list of some common game changers and how they tend to affect people's eating and activity, as well as a few strategies for dealing with them. If you know that one of these game changers is coming up for you, try creating a plan now using the information and tips from Chapters 7 and 8.

Wedding – Wedding planning can become a full-time job on its own, so time you once had for preparing meals or exercising might be replaced with meeting florists and photographers. However, getting married can be a strong motivator for people to look their best. Investing in a "Bride/Groom-to-be" exercise or nutrition program can be worth it. If getting married also means moving in with your spouse, you may also have to deal with a change in living arrangements (see next page).

Death of a Relative or Close Friend – A family member or friend's death can have multiple impacts: psychological, social and physical. Losing someone close to you may cause stress, sadness and depression, which can all manifest as less-than-ideal eating and physical activity decisions. Take time to mourn their loss. But you must also recognize that your life goes on and should be as healthy as possible. If this person prepared your meals for you, you may have to start cooking on your own. If this person motivated you to stay active, then the drive needs to come from someone else; possibly from within yourself. If this person helped you get through tough times, you'll have to find alternate ways to cope with stress. After grieving, focusing on healthy changes is one of the most uplifting actions you can take: exercise has been shown to fight depression just as well as medication. Live your best, healthiest life in memory of those you care about most.

Disease or Injury – Getting sick or injured is a bummer. You're usually less physically active during these times, so your healthy eating habits become even more important. If you're burning fewer calories, then you need to consume fewer calories. You can eat more often and include more fruits and veggies, so you feel like you're getting food when you want it without consuming excess calories. On the other hand, injury or sickness may also mean you have more time available to prepare healthy meals or exercise a non-injured area of the body. If you were injured while exercising, consider hiring a trainer for awhile to make sure that you get into an exercise routine that won't hurt you again. It's about moving better…and then moving more.

Job, Career or Work Hours Change – The daily routine is really important to us humans – we're creatures of habit. That's why this book is focused on making small, positive adjustments to existing habits. Changes like a new job, job loss or change in your working hours, however, can cause major upheaval in your daily routine. These changes can lead to high levels of stress and less healthy decisions. But this can also be a time when habits are changed for the better, not worse.

If you know the job change is coming, make a plan for maintaining or improving your current eating and physical activity habits; then test it out and adjust as necessary. Being prepared makes the transition much easier. If the change is abrupt, focus on minimizing any new stress this has caused. Then create a revised plan and strategies based on your new demands at work. For example, if you have more time due to being laid off, review your Whys – can you become more physically active now that you have the time? It'll actually improve the job search process by keeping you positive and focused. If you have less time because you've gotten longer work hours or a longer commute, check your list of commitments; is there anything else that you can move off your plate so that your health remains a priority?

New Child – Having or adopting a child is a wonderful, yet very stressful period in your life. In the beginning, every single aspect of life is impacted, from sleep to schedule. Being sleep deprived is an added stressor, so finding ways to cope with this situation is essential. Create a plan. If you're off from work for a period of time, you may have to refocus your Easy Eight Habit strategies toward being at home.

Having a support system is crucial for prioritizing your health. See if you can create a schedule with your significant other, friend, family member or a daycare center where you get some "me" time every day. An hour a day where you can work out, go for a walk, cook a healthy meal or even take a nap! Then you can return refreshed, renewed and ready to return the favor. The more you take care of yourself, the better parent and role model you can be.

Moving or Change in Living Arrangements – This can be a positive or negative event depending on what situation you are moving into. Are you living with roommates who can be a part of your support system, as workout or cooking buddies? Are you moving in with a significant other who you can split chores or meal preparation with? Will you have access to a better or worse kitchen? Will you be close to a gym or other exercise facility? Is the neighborhood a physical activity-friendly place – are there parks, sidewalks, bike lanes?

Moving in with my girlfriend (now wife), Becca, has made me even healthier. She takes her sleep seriously, so I quickly found myself going from six hours of sleep a night to seven or more. And she starts most mornings by blending up a green smoothie with ingredients like kale or parsley with apples, pears or grapefruit, water and ice. I began having these smoothies regularly once we started living together. As a result, I've significantly increased my fruit and veggie intake.

Divorce – The end of a marriage can be a difficult time, especially if children are involved. There may be extra demands on your time and your finances both during and after the divorce process. The efficiencies of living as a couple may no longer be there, so you may have to do the laundry, wash dishes, go to work and take care of a child by yourself. Assess your new schedule and available time: can you maintain your current eating and physical activity habits? Or do you have to adjust them? If one habit is going to become harder, can you make up for it by improving another Easy Eight Habit? Or rescheduling other demands?

Additionally, the person you're separating from may have had a big influence on your lifestyle. Think about the role your soon-to-be-ex played in your diet and exercise routines. If it was a negative influence, then you may be in for a boost. But if the influence was positive, you need to start looking for alternate sources of motivation and accountability to stay focused on living well – like family, friends or colleagues. If you're not sure what kind of effect the relationship had on your lifestyle, remember your habits before you two met…that may be a first clue to how your habits can change for the better.

Graduation or Retirement (aka Graduating from your career) – Graduations often kick off significant transitions in responsibility and routines, whether you're graduating from high school, college or are at the end of your career. Look through your current habits and anticipate how graduation will change them. If you were on a sports team or had an active job, then a fair amount of exercise may be removed from your routine. On the flipside, if this is the first time you can make it to the gym in a decade, that's a good thing.

From a nutrition perspective, you need to assess where and how you will be getting your food in the future. Will you be eating more at home? At work? Or will you be moving away from home and living on a campus that has all-you-can-eat dining halls? Do you need to start grocery shopping? The sooner you can adjust your habits to reflect your updated schedule, the more likely you are to maintain or improve your results.

Change in Financial Situation – Whether it's getting a raise, losing a job, buying a home or having a child, many major life events result in a shift in income or expenses. We're all used to living at a certain comfort level, depending on our current resources. If these resources increase, you may be able to enlist additional sources of support and guidance such as a trainer, dietitian and coach.

On the other hand, if your resources go down, you may have to adjust your expectations. But rather than immediately cut the funds devoted to your physical activity and eating habits, re-examine your budget and see if other purchases are more expendable. Compared to a lot of other "toys," staying active and eating well provides a long-term return to those who choose to invest in it: greater independence as you age, better health and richer experiences. If income does become a major concern for aspects of your life beyond the "extras," there are plenty of low-cost opportunities to eat well and stay active: working out in parks, going for a jog, finding a discount gym, enlisting support from friends or family, reading books on fitness and nutrition (free from the library) and bulk cooking at home. Any of these ideas provide a big, healthy bang for your buck.

Leaving a Sport – Many athletes are able to eat whatever they want while competing – pizza, pasta and cookies – because they burn off the calories through daily practices and games. However, these same athletes, whether they played in high school, college or professionally, are at risk of gaining weight soon after they leave their sport. If your physical activity habits decrease but your eating habits stay the same, then you'll likely gain weight. Unfortunately, many athletes are not prepared for this transition, so they continue to eat the way they always have and slowly watch the pounds pile on. Becoming aware of this situation is the first step to combating it.

While a lot of former athletes stay active after leaving their sport, most don't return to the level of their competitive days. Your body will require some time to downgrade its demand for food, however, since it was used to operating at high levels of food intake and calorie burn for years. For this reason, focus on improving nutrient density (Habit #3), maintaining or increasing meal frequency (Habit #1) and only slightly reducing portion sizes (Habit #2). The goal of this transition is to eat better (more nutrients, fewer calories), not to eat less.

CONCLUSION: THE CLIMB HAS BEGUN

You may be reaching the end of the journey contained within this book, but this is just the beginning of a lifelong process of health, fitness, weight and lifestyle improvement. I hope that you've found a number of the activities, questions and ideas useful in helping you flip the switch, push the spring and create a solution that works for *you* based on the Easy Eight Habits. I hope you have a crowd cheering you on, both internally and externally, as you start your ascent to the top of your mountain: your Whys.

The path to success is rarely a straight shot to the top. You will stumble, you will get frustrated and you'll have periods of self-doubt. It's all a part of the process. But taking consistent action, paired with the ability to reassess, adjust and integrate feedback as you go, will set you on a path that *will* get you to the summit – even if it takes a few switchbacks. Don't believe in any one approach; just believe in yourself.

I also hope that this is not the last time you'll read this book. I encourage you to revisit it as you grow and change from your experiences, as the words written here may take on new meanings. Tips that didn't work for you previously may be useful in the future. Some activities you chose not to do may seem like a good idea later on. My goal is for this book to be an asset to you today, tomorrow and for the rest of your life.

If you want to live your best life from now on, then there's no reason to wait for tomorrow. Right now is the right time in your life to start or continue making the positive changes that will get you to your health, fitness and weight goals, which will lead to the life you want and deserve to have.

It's been an awesome journey so far and I hope you will join me. Please share your successes, frustrations and questions with me: **info@jasonmachowsky.com**.

I look forward to hearing from you!

EPILOGUE

THE NINTH HABIT

The Ninth Habit doesn't involve making a specific change to your physical activity or eating habits. Instead it has to do with thinking better. The aim of the Ninth Habit is to create an internal belief that no matter what happens, you can and will live the life you want – including staying active and eating well. Taking action on the Ninth Habit means motivating your subconscious to work for you, rather than against you.

In their book *Switch*, Chip and Dan Heath create a fantastic metaphor for how we make decisions. Our brain is like an elephant and its rider. Our logical, conscious mind is the rider who, by using his "reins" of logic, can pull the elephant in the direction he wants it to go. On the other hand, the elephant is our subconscious, which represents our inner desires, emotions and feelings. The elephant, as we know, ultimately has the power in the relationship because it can choose to go wherever the heck it wants…and take the rider along for the ride! Just insert a mouse (fear) or a tempting patch of grasses and fruits (the elephant's favorite foods) or any other event that causes an emotional response. But the rider does all he can to stay in control, and through effort and training can retain control for quite some time.

Two situations will cause us to run into trouble:

First, a strong scare or temptation can make the elephant completely override the rider, despite all of his efforts. For example, think back to a time when you had a strong food craving or temptation that made you "lose control."

Second, our logical rider can exhaust his energy by constantly making the elephant perform tasks it does not really want to do. The rider knows these activities need to get done, so he forces the elephant to do them by using lots of effort and control, which can be tiring! After a while, the rider gets tired and the elephant gets mad; so the elephant starts rebelling and going where it wants. Where your elephant wants to go is what matters most.

For example, imagine spending a long day at school or work doing things that you don't really want to do. You're using all of your rider's control and energy to get yourself to do the tasks that you know you need to do. By the end of the day, your rider is exhausted and is at the mercy of the elephant – your subconscious feelings.

Now imagine it's 6 PM and you have to decide whether to go to the gym for a workout or just go home, watch TV and have some chips. If the elephant is truly motivated to go to the gym, you will go. But if it would rather just go home and have some chips, the rider is too tired to force the elephant to lace up its sneakers. Imagine yourself in that situation right now: are you on the gym elephant or the chips elephant?

As you can see, the subconscious elephant plays a crucial role in our ability to achieve and maintain a healthy lifestyle. Why? Because the subconscious is what's responsible for our hunches, gut reactions, fears, temptations, emotional reactions and everything else that we do even though it doesn't "make sense" to us. Why do we do things that we *know* are not good for us? Often because they make us *feel* better, at least temporarily. We're being influenced by feelings, not logic. Here's Maya Angelou's insight: "I've learned that people will forget what you said, people will forget what you did, but people will never forget how you made them feel."

Not only is the elephant ultimately more powerful than the rider, it's also taking in and processing a whole lot more information than the rider is aware of. Michael Gelb, author of *How to Think Like Leonardo da Vinci*, writes "Brain researchers estimate that your unconscious database outweighs the conscious on an order exceeding ten million to one." And according to developmental biologist Dr. Bruce Lipton, the subconscious mind can process data almost *one million times* faster than the conscious mind. So we need to be sending our subconscious mind information and feedback that drives it toward achieving our goals and desires rather than away from them. Otherwise, it's you versus an elephant.

So how do you win over the elephant onto your side of the battle? Be persistent and be positive.

PART 1: BE PERSISTENT

STAY THE COURSE

Robert Collier, an American motivational author from the early 1900s, wrote "Success is the sum of small efforts, repeated day in and day out." That's why you need to celebrate success in all of its forms, big and small! Don't forget that maintaining good habits is a success; new commitments, challenges and concerns come up all the time, and success means persevering through this constant flux while doing what you need to do to get results. That's why you have your Whys, Easy Eight Habits and strategies—they are the rock you can focus on amidst a life filled with change.

Staying the course means:

- Committing to going after your health, fitness or weight change desires, Whys and chosen Easy Eight Habits wholeheartedly.

- Putting in the practice and effort required to get better at your chosen Easy Eight Habit, such as learning how to cook or count calories, how to exercise safely, how to read ingredient lists and food labels, or skim restaurant menus for the best options.

- Accepting any slipups you make and focusing on the next workout or the next meal rather than blaming, making excuses or waiting until "tomorrow" or "Monday" to start being healthy again.

- Keeping records of your progress via assessments and evaluations to build momentum on previous successes and as a tool for improvement when dealing with challenges.

- Believing in persistence over giving up, whether you're one yard or one hundred yards from the goal line.

STUCK? DON'T ASSUME – ASK.

According to my fifth-grade teacher, when you ASS-U-ME, you make an ass out of you and me. So don't assume that anything is too complicated or too challenging. You can always ask and get answers – hopefully, the answers that will let you move forward.

A great example: if you're new to the gym and have never used exercise equipment, don't assume that they're only for mechanical geniuses, meatheads or fitness nuts. Ask a knowledgeable member, or better yet ask a trainer! Investing in a trainer for a few sessions to learn the basics will pay dividends for the rest of your life. You'll become more self-sufficient with exercise and you'll reduce your risk of injury – all from asking for help rather than giving up.

TOUGH OUT THE BEGINNINGS

How will you know if you're still learning and improving? You'll feel uncomfortable. Remember Marshall Thurber's quote, "Anything worth doing well is worth doing badly at first." And usually doing something badly feels frustrating or uncomfortable.

Imagine kids learning to ride a bike. They get on and start moving. They may swerve and fall. If you compared them to Tour de France racers, well then, the kids would be downright awful. But we don't do that! We realize that they're learning, so we motivate them to continue to get better. They get back up on the bike, get a little straighter, fall a little bit less and improve until they can ride as straight as an arrow.

We need to treat our attempts to make positive changes the same way, and that means giving ourselves permission to make mistakes or look silly.

A personal example: I never learned how to ride a bike as a kid. I tried learning a few times as a late teen, but I was always self-conscious and worried about what others would think. So I made half-hearted attempts on my friends' driveways and usually quit after fifteen minutes. Then finally in the summer of 2011, I was with my wife Becca and I realized that biking was an activity we could enjoy doing together for the rest of our lives both locally and when traveling.

I chose to stop worrying about how I looked. We rented bikes and I set myself up in the relatively empty parking lot of a hotel. Yep, people saw me. Yep, I looked ridiculous for quite a while (and I still do a bit), but I didn't care, and at the age of 28 I learned how to ride a bike. Amazingly I was actually zipping around after an hour or so, though when a car came within ten feet of me I freaked out. I've still got a ways to go, but I'm working at it!

Similarly, your first home-cooked, healthy meal may not taste gourmet and your first workout or dance lesson may not make you feel like you're a pro. But just like with any other new skill or ability, the more you practice, the better you'll get. And the better you get, the more confident and efficient you become. And then what was once uncomfortable becomes easy.

When this happens, look back with pride at what you've accomplished. Give yourself a pat on the back. Then push yourself to do or learn a little more – continuous growth means staying a little bit uncomfortable.

PART TWO: BE POSITIVE

Staying positive can become a daily challenge when you're bombarded with negative thoughts all the time, from friends, family, co-workers and even the eleven 'o clock news. It's important, though, because your outlook on life can impact your commitment to living healthier.

Here's a list of some of the best ideas I've seen for creating positive responses to negative situations. With enough practice, you can start automatically responding positively to most events, good and bad. In Monty Python terms, it's called "Always Look on the Bright Side of Life."

VISUALIZE SUCCESS

Visualization is an applied meditation where you focus your mind on a particular result. In your case, picture yourself successfully taking action on your Easy Eight Habit, executing your strategies and achieving your Whys. Visualization is "planning" for your subconscious – then the elephant, along with the rider of your conscious mind, can help you get to your Whys.

It's not fluff; this stuff works. And a little goes a long way. Ten minutes of visualization can save you up to seventy minutes of wasted effort. How the heck is this possible? Visualization works on your subconscious by activating your Reticular Activating System, which builds motivation and increases your awareness of better and healthier options around you. Your subconscious will start filtering the hundreds of thousands of stimuli that your mind receives every day on its own.

Think about how many things you can sense right now, in this moment, let alone the entire day: sight, sound, smell, taste, touch. Too much to actively think about! But that's why you have a subconscious. From these stimuli, the subconscious will start looking for the answers to your visualizations on its own and then draw your conscious attention to it. In other words, the elephant is actually helping lead itself!

You could become aware of restaurants with healthier options near your workplace. You may strike up a conversation with a friend, colleague or stranger about eating better that leads to a new support system. You may go down a new supermarket aisle and find some healthy foods that you love to eat. You might start focusing more on all of the healthy decisions you made during the day rather than getting down on yourself for having eaten two small cookies late in the afternoon. Visualization streamlines your mind's thoughts into action, and ultimately results.

The key to getting your subconscious onboard is to fuel these visualizations with images and emotion. Strong emotion is inextricably linked with your memories. Do you remember what you did three years ago on March 16th? If you can and it's not your birthday, that's impressive. On the other hand, how much can you remember about the day JFK was assassinated, 9/11/2001, or your wedding day? Most of us can probably remember what was going on those days, even extremely small details. How we felt, what we did, everything.

That's why it's so important to create strong, motivating Whys and clear, detailed strategies for your Easy Eight Habits. Then spend five to ten minutes each day with your eyes closed etching these motivations and actions into your mind so you can see, feel, hear, smell and even taste yourself doing them in your mind. You can even create a tangible visual; for example, if you always wanted to confidently take your shirt off at the beach, photo-shop your face onto the body that you want and add it to a beach scene. That's a visual of you achieving what you want.

You want symbols of success to be so strong in your mind that you can just close your eyes and see them. With the backing of strong emotion, success is no longer an "if"—it's a matter of when!

LOVE THE PROCESS

A simple, yet very powerful concept: You enjoy the things you enjoy. If you love skiing, I bet you can't wait until the winter's first big snow. If you love golf, I'm sure you are just counting the days until the next time you are on the course. You wake up excited to do what you love. So, find the healthy eating and activity habits that you love to do – healthy foods you look forward to eating, exercise that's fun. It's a system of trial-and-error, and that's why you need to love the process. It's experimenting. It's playing detective. It's about keeping score. Sounds a lot more interesting than "eat more fruit and vegetables," right? You're taking the same actions, but thinking about them differently.

FEEL IT FROM THE INSIDE OUT

Jobs change, friends move away, life events happen, but in the end, the one person that will always be around you is…you. The only way you can ensure you'll maintain a healthy lifestyle no matter what happens is to create an internal desire to keep doing the right thing, and a positive outlook that comes from yourself rather than from external factors.

The best way to feel positive from the inside out? Smile. Do it more, do it for no reason. Think of funny jokes. Call a friend. Hug someone that you love. Think of a great experience you had recently. One of the quickest, surefire ways to feel better: laugh. Try it! Smile and laugh for fifteen seconds straight and see how you feel after; you can force the laugh if you need to. Not only will you find it to be a good abdominal workout, you'll probably feel better too.

LEAN ON YOUR STRENGTHS AND SUCCESSES AS YOU IMPROVE

Make a list of your strengths and past successes. This will help you in a number of ways:

- To be optimistic about your chances of success, when you realize that you have strengths that you can use on your health, fitness or weight change journey.

- To realize that you've already taken a number of positive steps towards reaching your Whys; you're already well on your way.

- To give you a list of strengths and successes that you can turn to when you get frustrated. It's always more productive to draw solutions from the positive rather than get stuck on the negative.

Many successful, powerful people, including CEOs, former athletes, politicians and celebrities, deal with health, fitness and weight issues. Just like you, they may not realize that the strengths they use in their careers – such as dedication, motivation, sociability, problem solving, action planning, organizing, inspiring others, etc. – are exactly what they need to solve their health issues. It's just that they've never considered using these strengths in other areas of their life, like improving their health or fitness.

Once you shift your focus this way, the process of making healthy changes becomes much clearer, and often much easier. It can still be challenging to eat better or become more active, but now you are approaching it with your strongest ideas and resources…the things you are good at!

MY STRENGTHS	MY PREVIOUS SUCCESSES IN ALL ASPECTS OF LIFE

LISTEN MORE

Has someone ever asked you for advice and then immediately done the complete opposite of what you suggested? Do you find that frustrating? Do you feel less likely to give that person advice in the future?

Some people can hear what you're saying—but they're not listening. Listening is more than just hearing. It's about being receptive to the information, understanding how it may be most beneficial to you and then choosing whether or not to take action based on that information. Developing your listening skills in three areas can improve your life, including your health and fitness:

Listening to Others – When someone is speaking to you, don't just hear the words they're saying; try to understand where they're coming from. Most advice is given by people who genuinely care about you and want to help – so resist the urge to get defensive.

If you've had friends, family members or others speak to you about your health in a concerned way, odds are they aren't just trying to nag you or make you mad. They love you, and they want you to be around and involved in their lives for a long, long time. If you feel that some people's comments place too much pressure on you, speak up! That's the only way they'll understand how *you* feel. Then they can adjust their message. When receiving advice, the best thing to do is:

- Thank them for the advice.

- Tell them how you found it interesting or useful for you, or why you feel it's not helpful for you.

- Tell them what steps you intend to make based on the advice.

- Then actually do it!

Listening to Yourself – You are your own biggest conversation partner, to the tune of about 50,000 internal mini-conversations per day. So if you want to have a positive outlook, those mini-conversations had better be positive and constructive. In addition, make sure you're listening to yourself physically. Fatigue, pain and stress are all warning signs. They indicate that something is wrong with your body, and that you must change some of your actions to improve it. If an exercise creates pain, stop doing it and learn the correct movements. If you're always tired, take stock of how much sleep you're getting and whether your meals are regular and balanced. By acknowledging your body and your thoughts, you become open and responsive to the very person who is most concerned about your well-being: you!

Listening to Your Intuition – Use your intuition to override the elephant. Remember, your subconscious can be working for you, telling you to steer clear of the "free food" area at work…or against you, telling you that you deserve that slice of pizza you just smelled because you had a long day at work. The key to listening to your intuition is:

1. Becoming aware of your subconscious and its influence on you.

2. Understanding the root of your subconscious urges. Is it stress? Is it motivation?

3. Making a thoughtful decision by carefully assessing your subconscious urge. Is it in line with your health, fitness or weight change desires and Whys?

If you're ever in doubt, your intuition is an excellent guide. ***If it doesn't feel right, don't do it.***

BE APPRECIATIVE AND UPLIFTING

I don't think I've ever seen someone get sad or mad from receiving a sincere compliment or thanks. Try these little things to add more sincere appreciation to your life, both for yourself and for the people who help you:

- Say please and thank you more.

- Recognize out loud the little things other people do for you.

- Pat yourself on the back when you have a success or use one of your strengths.

- Aim to give at least five compliments a day, the more specific the better: "I really appreciate how you cook dinner on the evenings I need to go to the gym," or "Thanks so much for always giving me helpful tips on my presentations; it really motivates me to do better each time."

- Write down two to three events or people that you're grateful for every day. Be as specific as possible. And thank them the following day!

PAY IT FORWARD

Start sharing your successes and lessons learned with others as soon as you can. Here are a few ways you can do that:

Read, reread and grow – Each time you read this book or other fitness, nutrition or wellness books, you'll gain more insights about your mindset, get new ideas for executing the Easy Eight Habits and better internalize your own commitment to a healthy, fulfilling lifestyle. Share these insights with others.

Teach others – Give a talk at your local community center, or mentor someone who wants to make positive changes to their eating or activity habits. Offer to show someone a new exercise that you know well or teach them how to cook a healthy meal. Not only will you help other people overcome their own barriers and challenges, you'll receive numerous rewards as well. Teaching builds your self-confidence, helps you clarify your own ideas, allows you to confront and correct your own inconsistencies and reinforces the healthy habits you are currently performing. Teaching will make walking the walk easier and much more fulfilling.

Help others – Be involved in someone's support system, Mastermind or community group for positive health changes. Lead by example. Inspire someone to go to the gym with you, or invite them over to try a healthy meal you'll both enjoy. By raising others up, you will feel and live better throughout all areas of life.

Give to others – Give a copy of a fitness or nutrition book to someone who is receptive to it. Lend or buy them this book! It doesn't have to be related to money or things, of course. Give your time, energy, effort and positivity and do so without expecting anything in return. You'll be surprised how much you get back in return when you actually need it. Just be sure to keep your own healthy lifestyle commitments as well!

YOUR PERSONAL 12-WEEK ACTION PLAN

These general guidelines will help you get the most from your 12-week action plan:

1. ***Try everything with an open mind, but know that everything is a "challenge by choice."*** All the activities in the book are designed to help you to grow and improve, not to be a source of stress. You can always skip an activity.

2. ***Continue to do what works best for you.*** Over the course of 12 weeks, you'll try a range of activities, assessments, evaluations and reflections aimed at different ways to improve your health. The idea is to expose you to lots of options and allow you to choose the ones that work best for you. If you find a particular strategy, activity, evaluation or action that works really well, feel free to continue it beyond the week that it's assigned. *You can download and print the Appendix forms in full size here: deathofthediet.com/forms*

3. ***Save all of your forms and evaluations, on paper or as computer documents.*** At the end of the 12 weeks, you'll have a chance to reflect on the whole experience. You'll be amazed at how much progress you've made, both physically and mentally, in three months. A "personal

journey and solution journal" documenting the journey can also serve as a roadmap to living your healthiest life possible. Continue to update it, and it will grow as you do.

WEEK 1 - WHY CHANGE?

- *Read:* Foreword and Chapters 1 through 3.

- *Action:* Sign your Pledge to start your journey toward wellness. Take a picture or make a copy of it and put it somewhere you'll see it every day. (Foreword, pg. 7) You can also download a copy of it here: deathofthediet.com/pledge

- *Reflect:* Define Your Whys, based on the Seven Dimensions of Wellness. (Chapter 3, pg. 24-26)

- *Action:* Write down your Whys on index cards or create a visual representation of your Whys, and place them in at least two places where you'll see them every day. (Chapter 3, pg. 31-32)

- *Assess:* Perform initial assessments to establish a baseline for tracking your progress over the next 12 weeks. If you choose to track any number-based measurements such as weight, waist circumference, clothing size, or body fat percentage, choose at least two so you can get multiple points of feedback. Sometimes a person's weight may not go down after the first few weeks of making changes, but their pants or dress size will decrease since muscle weighs more, but takes up less space, than fat. Also aim to include at least one feelings-based assessment, such as hunger, energy or stress levels. These assessments often improve before numbers-based assessments and let you know you're on the right track. They also shine a light on the long-term sustainability of your chosen Easy Eight Habit changes.

- *Connect:* When you feel comfortable, share your Whys with a loved one or friend that you trust.

WEEK 2 - UNDERSTANDING THE PROCESS OF CHANGE

- *Read:* Chapters 4 through 6.

- *Reflect:* If you've tried any diets in the past, do the Chronic Dieting Insight Activity. (Chapter 4, pg. 38-39)

- *Reflect:* If you're not doing the Chronic Dieting Insight Activity, take notes on your previous attempts at "pushing the spring" for improving your eating or physical activity habits: what worked and what didn't? (Chapter 4, pg. 39)

- *Reflect:* Take notes describing your current comfort zone (where your spring is), how that came to be your normal routine (what put the spring where it is) and how you can start slowly pushing the spring forward for results. (Chapter 4, pg. 37-40)

- *Read & Reflect:* In Chapter 7, skim the Rationales, Assessments and Recommended Changes for all of the Easy Eight Habits. Choose the Easy Eight Habit that you feel is most realistic and achievable for you.

WEEK 3 - CREATING YOUR PLAN

- *Read:* The first part of Chapter 8 on Creating Plans, Strategies and Evaluations. (pg. 163-180)

- *Assess:* Perform your chosen Easy Eight Habit assessment for at least three days, preferably seven. (Chapter 7, pages based on your Habit)

- *Read & Reflect:* Read the Strategies section of your chosen Easy Eight Habit again, and take notes on the ideas for action that you like best (Chapter 7, pages based on your Habit). Why do those actions in particular appeal to you?

- *Action:* Create an action plan for your Habit using your own ideas and the Easy Eight Strategies Worksheet in the Appendix. Come up with at least three actions you can take to work your chosen Easy Eight Habit into your life. You can categorize them as "at home," "at work," "over the weekend," etc.

- *Reflect:* Define and write down your sources of motivation (Chapter 8, pg. 168).

WEEK 4 - TAKING ACTION

- *Action - Habit 1, Week 1:* Start carrying out the action plan for your chosen Easy Eight Habit, using your ideas from Week 3.

- *Evaluate:* Track the effects of your actions using an Evaluation form; evaluate your progress based on the feedback you believe will be most beneficial for you (Chapter 8, pg. 174-177). Also feel free to use any additional journals you feel are appropriate. (Appendix)

- *Read:* The second half of Chapter 8 on creating support systems. (pg. 181-196)

- *Action:* Create your positive and negative people lists. (Chapter 8, pg. 185)

- *Connect:* Reach out and start building your support list. (Chapter 8, pg. 187)

- *Connect:* Begin publicizing your changes based on how comfortable you feel about it. (Chapter 8, pg. 181-183)

WEEK 5 - GETTING A LITTLE HELP FROM YOUR FRIENDS

- *Action & Evaluate - Habit 1, Week 2:* Continue to track the effects of your chosen Easy Eight Habit change using your personalized Evaluation form.

- *Read:* Chapter 9.

- *Action:* Start using the "Roadblock - Negative to Positive Response Feedback Form." (Chapter 9, pg. 206)

- *Connect:* Continue to build your support system and publicize as you feel ready. (Chapter 8)

- *Connect:* Begin asking for guidance and feedback from your Support System. (Chapter 8, pg. 192-195)

- *Connect:* If you'd like to, look for a mentor or Mastermind/community group. Feel free to use someone from your support system list. (Chapter 8, pg. 188-192)

WEEK 6 - SELF-ORGANIZATION WEEK

- *Action & Evaluate - Habit 1, Week 3:* Continue to track the progress of your chosen Easy Eight Habit change using your personalized Evaluation form.

- *Evaluation Extra:* Every night this week, write down your three biggest to-dos for the next day on your daily Evaluation form, and then keep the list with you the following day. (Chapter 8, pg. 175)

- *Reflect & Action:* Re-read Chapter 7 with more attention to detail, and choose the two other Habits that you feel most confident in pursuing. Then brainstorm and write down at least three ideas for taking action on each by using the Easy Eight Strategies Worksheet. You'll have two weeks to brainstorm on an action plan, since you begin improving your second Habit in Week 8.

- *Action:* Write down and read through your commitments. Then perform the 4 D's activity to get them streamlined. (Chapter 9, pg. 212)

- *Action:* Fill Out Healthy Food Preference List (Appendix)

WEEK 7 - OPERATION: HEALTH WEEK

- *Action & Evaluate - Habit 1, Week 4:* Continue to track the results of your chosen Easy Eight Habit change using your personalized Evaluation form. At this point, this action may have become a habit. So when you start establishing a new Habit next week, this one should be easy to continue.

- *Assess:* Based on your Chapter 7 reflection from last week, choose the next Easy Eight Habit that you feel will be easiest for you, and perform that Habit's assessment for at least three days, preferably seven (Chapter 7, page based on your Habit).

- *Read:* Epilogue: The Ninth Habit.

- *Reflect:* Think about elements of your life that may be impacting your ability to make positive eating or physical activity changes – like smoking, inadequate sleep, chronic stress, etc. Brainstorm and write down ways to make improvements to these situations, like getting one more hour of sleep a night, smoking two fewer cigarettes per day, doing ten minutes of breathing or visualization exercises daily, etc. (Chapter 9, pg. 209-211)

- *Action:* Schedule any checkups you need to ensure you're healthy inside and out. (Ch 9. pg. 214-216)

- *Action:* Try a new fruit or vegetable from the Healthy Food Preference List and update the list to show whether you like it or not. ***Note when trying new foods:** You may have to try a new food a few times to develop a taste for it, so if you don't totally hate the food the first time around, try it a few more times. You could also combine the new food with familiar foods. For example, if you're trying to integrate brown rice into your routine, try mixing half brown and half white with your usual dinner and gradually increase the amount of brown rice served each meal.*

WEEK 8 - PERSISTENCE WEEK

- *Action & Evaluate - Habit 2, Week 1:* Start making changes to your second chosen Easy Eight Habit based on your ideas from Weeks 6 and 7. Track the progress of your chosen Easy Eight Habit change using your personalized Evaluation form. Feel free to adjust the Evaluation form based on the new Habit, if that helps you. Remember to continue performing your first Habit as well, which should hopefully be much easier to do on a daily and weekly basis than when you first started – ideally, it'll require very little extra thought or effort, since it's now a regular part of your routine.

- *Action & Evaluation Extra:* Perform one additional unplanned physical activity daily (see Chapter 7, pg. 154-156 and 159-160, for examples such as walking the stairs instead of taking the elevator) or one extra day of exercise this week (Habit #6) and write down what it was in your personalized Evaluation form.

- *Reflect:* Spend five minutes daily visualizing your Whys, and notice how that time impacts your stress, energy and ability to make positive decisions the rest of the day. (Chapter 3, pg. 31, Chapter 9, pg. 210 and Epilogue, pg. 228-229)

- *Reflect & Action:* Choose a food or exercise skill you'd like to start developing or improve upon, and buy a book, take a class or try another action to learn how to do it. Write down what skill you'll be developing on your Evaluation form. (Epilogue, pg. 226-227)

- *Reflect & Action:* Read through the "Game Changers" list and start preparing an action plan for any Game Changers you foresee occurring within the next three months. (Chapter 9, pg. 216-221)

- *Action:* Try a new grain or lean protein from the Healthy Food Preference List and update the list to indicate whether you like it or not.

WEEK 9 - POSITIVITY WEEK

- *Action & Evaluate - Habit 2, Week 2:* Continue to track the effects of your chosen Easy Eight Habit change using your personalized Evaluation form.

- *Evaluation Extra:* Every day write down three things you're grateful for, either in general or from that day, on your daily Evaluation form. Be as specific as possible about who, what, why, etc. (Epilogue, pg. 233)

- *Evaluation Extra:* Every day write down two to three successes you achieved that day, no matter how big or small, on your daily Evaluation form. The successes can be from any aspect of life or health. (Chapter 8, pg. 175-176)

- *Action:* Fill out your Strengths and Previous Successes List. At the end of the week, add on the successes you listed on your daily Evaluation forms and any more strengths you realize you've developed. (Epilogue, pg. 231)

- *Reflect:* If you're dealing with any recurring negative thoughts about yourself or your ability to make positive habit changes, try this: Imagine one of your closest family members or best friends came to you with the same issue and negative thoughts you're having – for example, "I can never stick to eating healthy, I always cheat at some point, so what's the use in trying?" What would you tell your close friend or relative? Write down the issue and your response. Now take that advice to heart for yourself.

- **Action:** Try a new fruit or vegetable from the Healthy Food Preference List and update the list to indicate whether you like it or not.

WEEK 10 - CONNECTION & FEEDBACK

- **Action & Evaluate - Habit 2, Week 3:** Continue to track the progress of your chosen Easy Eight Habit change using your personalized Evaluation form.

- **Assess:** Based on your Chapter 7 reflection from Week 6, choose the third Easy Eight Habit you feel will be easiest for you, and perform that Habit's assessment for at least three days, preferably seven (Chapter 7, page based on your Habit). If you've already chosen two eating habits, try a physical activity habit this time. And vice versa.

- **Connect & Evaluation Extra:** Praise or thank two to three people each day: tell them what you appreciate about their efforts or what they mean to you and your life. Write down their names, their relationship to you and what you praised them for in your daily Evaluation form. (Epilogue, pg. 233)

- **Connect & Reflect:** Ask for Feedback from two to three people in your Support System. Write down the insights you learn from them, and then take any actions that stem from their feedback. (Chapter 8 pg. 192-195, Chapter 9, pg. 206-209)

- **Connect:** Over the course of the week, call, email or Skype three people you've been meaning to get in touch with for a while. If you feel comfortable, you can also tell them about your healthy lifestyle changes. Write down the three people, when you contacted them and what you discussed on your daily Evaluation form. (Chapter 8, pg. 181-182)

- *Action:* Try a new grain or lean protein from the Healthy Food Preference List and update the list to indicate whether you like it or not.

WEEK 11 - PAY IT FORWARD

- *Action & Evaluate - Habit 3, Week 1:* Start making changes to your third chosen Easy Eight Habit based on the ideas you created in Weeks 6 and 7. Track the results of your Habit change using your personalized Evaluation form. Feel free to adjust the Evaluation form based on the new Habit. Remember to continue performing your first and second Habits as well – they should both be part of your regular routine now.

- *Action & Evaluation Extra:* Pay it forward to yourself by pushing a little bit harder: Perform one additional unplanned physical activity daily (see Chapter 7, pg. 154-156 and 159-160, for examples such as walking the stairs instead of taking the elevator) or one extra day of exercise this week (Habit #6) and write down what it was in your personalized Evaluation form.

- *Reflect:* Create a list of how you want to start paying it forward, or any particular people you want to pay it forward to. How will you contact them, and what will you do? (Epilogue, pg. 233-234)

- *Action:* Three times this week, teach others some of the knowledge and skills you've gained over the past ten weeks. You can give a talk at a local organization, show your kids or family, share with a friend looking to make a positive change or write about your experience for the local newspaper. Write down how it went on your daily Evaluation form. (Chapter 8, pg. 181-182, Epilogue pg. 233-234)

- *Read:* Get back into the book and review any sections that you'd like to brush up on. Explore the book with a friend or family member. Learning and improving never ends. (Epilogue, pg. 233-234)

- *Action:* Try a new fruit or vegetable from the Healthy Food Preference List and update the list to indicate whether you like it or not.

WEEK 12 - REVIEW AND REFLECT

- *Action & Evaluate - Habit 3, Week 2:* Continue to track the progress of your chosen Easy Eight Habit change using your personalized Evaluation form.

- *Assess:* Revisit the assessments you chose in Week #1, or any assessments you may have switched to during to 12 weeks. Be sure to reassess both the number-based and the feeling-based factors.

- *Reflect:* Now that you've been carrying out action plans for a few months, spend five to ten minutes every day reading through your daily evaluations – look for patterns of positive results or improvement opportunities. Write them down and update your "Strengths and Successes" and "Roadblock" worksheets. (Chapter 9, pg. 206, Epilogue, pg. 231)

- *Reflect:* Revisit your Whys (Chapter 3, pg. 33). Do your motivations to change from three months ago still apply to the person you are today? Or have they changed based on how you've changed? Update your Whys and action plans if you need to.

- *Connect:* Contact someone that cares about you deeply. Tell them you're close to completing a 12-week action plan towards improving your health and wellbeing. Tell them about your experiences, feelings, hopes and action plans.

- *Reflect:* Think about how you'll continue improving once you complete this book: What books will you read? Will you hire a nutrition or fitness professional? Write down exactly who, what, where, when, how much, etc.

- *Action:* Try a new grain or lean protein from the Healthy Food Preference List and update the list to indicate whether you like it or not.

APPENDIX

- *Forms, Assessments and Journals*
- *Greens Recipes*
- *Mediator Release Test (MRT) and Lifestyle Eating and Performance (LEAP) Therapy Links*
- *Books and Programs for Making Positive Changes in All Seven Dimensions of Wellness*
- *Professional Coaching Services and Links*

FORMS, ASSESSMENTS AND JOURNALS

All forms can be downloaded for free from:

http://deathofthediet.com/forms/

Healthy Food Preference List

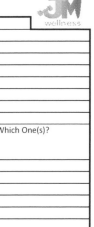

Grains/Starches				
Oatmeal	Like	Dislike	Never Tried	
Cream of Wheat	Like	Dislike	Never Tried	
Cream of Rice	Like	Dislike	Never Tried	
Grits	Like	Dislike	Never Tried	
Puffed kamut	Like	Dislike	Never Tried	
Puffed millet	Like	Dislike	Never Tried	
Cheerios	Like	Dislike	Never Tried	
Shredded Wheat	Like	Dislike	Never Tried	
Other Whole Grain Cereal without added sugar, marshmallows, etc.	Like	Dislike	Never Tried	Which One(s)?
Rye	Like	Dislike	Never Tried	
Spelt	Like	Dislike	Never Tried	
Amaranth	Like	Dislike	Never Tried	
Buckwheat	Like	Dislike	Never Tried	
Barley	Like	Dislike	Never Tried	
Quinoa	Like	Dislike	Never Tried	
Brown or Wild Rice	Like	Dislike	Never Tried	
Whole Wheat Pasta	Like	Dislike	Never Tried	
Whole Wheat Cous Cous	Like	Dislike	Never Tried	
Other Whole Grains	Like	Dislike	Never Tried	Which One(s)?
Whole Grain Breads/Rolls (i.e. Rye, Pumpernickel, Whole Wheat, Spelt, Millet, Rice)	Like	Dislike	Never Tried	Which One(s)?
Corn Tortillas	Like	Dislike	Never Tried	
Rice Tortialls	Like	Dislike	Never Tried	
Spelt Tortillas	Like	Dislike	Never Tried	
Potatoes	Like	Dislike	Never Tried	
Sweet Potatoes	Like	Dislike	Never Tried	
Yams	Like	Dislike	Never Tried	
Rice Cakes	Like	Dislike	Never Tried	
Corn	Like	Dislike	Never Tried	
Peas	Like	Dislike	Never Tried	
Black Beans	Like	Dislike	Never Tried	
Red Kidney Beans	Like	Dislike	Never Tried	
White Beans	Like	Dislike	Never Tried	
Garbanzo Beans	Like	Dislike	Never Tried	
Soybeans/Edamame	Like	Dislike	Never Tried	
Lentils	Like	Dislike	Never Tried	
Snacks:				
Granola Bars	Like	Dislike	Never Tried	
Popcorn	Like	Dislike	Never Tried	
Graham/Animal Crackers	Like	Dislike	Never Tried	

Green Vegetables:				Red Vegetables			
Alfalfa Sprouts	Like	Dislike	Never Tried	Beets	Like	Dislike	Never Tried
Arugula	Like	Dislike	Never Tried	Red Peppers	Like	Dislike	Never Tried
Artichokes	Like	Dislike	Never Tried	Radishes	Like	Dislike	Never Tried
Arugula	Like	Dislike	Never Tried	Radicchio	Like	Dislike	Never Tried
Asparagus	Like	Dislike	Never Tried	Red Onions	Like	Dislike	Never Tried
Beet Greens	Like	Dislike	Never Tried	Red Potatoes	Like	Dislike	Never Tried
Bok Choy	Like	Dislike	Never Tried	Rhubarb	Like	Dislike	Never Tried
Broccoflower	Like	Dislike	Never Tried	Tomatoes	Like	Dislike	Never Tried
Broccoli	Like	Dislike	Never Tried				
Broccoli Rabe	Like	Dislike	Never Tried				
Brussels Sprouts	Like	Dislike	Never Tried	Yellow/Orange Vegetables:			
Chicory	Like	Dislike	Never Tried	Yellow Beets	Like	Dislike	Never Tried
Chinese Cabbage	Like	Dislike	Never Tried	Butternut Squash	Like	Dislike	Never Tried
Chives	Like	Dislike	Never Tried	Carrots	Like	Dislike	Never Tried
Collard Greens	Like	Dislike	Never Tried	Yellow Peppers	Like	Dislike	Never Tried
Green Beans	Like	Dislike	Never Tried	Yellow Potatoes	Like	Dislike	Never Tried
Green Cabbage	Like	Dislike	Never Tried	Pumpkin	Like	Dislike	Never Tried
Celery	Like	Dislike	Never Tried	Rutabagas	Like	Dislike	Never Tried
Chayote Squash	Like	Dislike	Never Tried	Sweet Corn	Like	Dislike	Never Tried
Cucumbers	Like	Dislike	Never Tried	Sweet Potatoes	Like	Dislike	Never Tried
Endive	Like	Dislike	Never Tried	Yellow Tomatoes	Like	Dislike	Never Tried
Leafy Greens	Like	Dislike	Never Tried	Yellow Squash	Like	Dislike	Never Tried
Leeks	Like	Dislike	Never Tried				
Lettuce	Like	Dislike	Never Tried				
Green Onions	Like	Dislike	Never Tried	White/Tan Vegetables:			
Okra	Like	Dislike	Never Tried	Cauliflower	Like	Dislike	Never Tried
Peas	Like	Dislike	Never Tried	Garlic	Like	Dislike	Never Tried
Green Peppers	Like	Dislike	Never Tried	Ginger	Like	Dislike	Never Tried
Snow Peas	Like	Dislike	Never Tried	Jerusalem Artichoke	Like	Dislike	Never Tried
Spinach	Like	Dislike	Never Tried	Jicama	Like	Dislike	Never Tried
Sugar Snap Peas	Like	Dislike	Never Tried	Kohlrabi	Like	Dislike	Never Tried
Watercress	Like	Dislike	Never Tried	Mushrooms	Like	Dislike	Never Tried
Kale	Like	Dislike	Never Tried	Onions	Like	Dislike	Never Tried
Green Pepper	Like	Dislike	Never Tried	Parsnips	Like	Dislike	Never Tried
Fennel	Like	Dislike	Never Tried	Potatoes	Like	Dislike	Never Tried
Escarole	Like	Dislike	Never Tried	Shallots	Like	Dislike	Never Tried
Beet Greens	Like	Dislike	Never Tried	Turnips	Like	Dislike	Never Tried
Scallions	Like	Dislike	Never Tried	White Corn	Like	Dislike	Never Tried
Swiss Chard	Like	Dislike	Never Tried				
Blue/Purple Vegetables:							
Black Olives	Like	Dislike	Never Tried	Eggplant	Like	Dislike	Never Tried
Purple Asparagus	Like	Dislike	Never Tried	Purple Endive	Like	Dislike	Never Tried
Purple Cabbage	Like	Dislike	Never Tried	Purple Peppers	Like	Dislike	Never Tried
Purple Carrots	Like	Dislike	Never Tried	Purple Potatoes	Like	Dislike	Never Tried
				Black Salsify	Like	Dislike	Never Tried

Green Fruits:				Red Fruits:			
Avocados	Like	Dislike	Never Tried	Red Apples	Like	Dislike	Never Tried
Green Apples	Like	Dislike	Never Tried	Blood Oranges	Like	Dislike	Never Tried
Green Grapes	Like	Dislike	Never Tried	Cherries	Like	Dislike	Never Tried
Honeydew	Like	Dislike	Never Tried	Cranberries	Like	Dislike	Never Tried
Kiwifruit	Like	Dislike	Never Tried	Red Grapes	Like	Dislike	Never Tried
Limes	Like	Dislike	Never Tried	Grapefruit	Like	Dislike	Never Tried
Green Peas	Like	Dislike	Never Tried	Red Pears	Like	Dislike	Never Tried
				Pomegranates	Like	Dislike	Never Tried
Yellow/Orange Fruits:				Raspberries	Like	Dislike	Never Tried
Yellow Apples	Like	Dislike	Never Tried	Strawberries	Like	Dislike	Never Tried
Apricots	Like	Dislike	Never Tried	Watermelon	Like	Dislike	Never Tried
Gooseberries	Like	Dislike	Never Tried				
Cantaloupe	Like	Dislike	Never Tried	**White/Tan Fruits:**			
Yellow Figs	Like	Dislike	Never Tried	Bananas	Like	Dislike	Never Tried
Grapefruit	Like	Dislike	Never Tried	Dates	Like	Dislike	Never Tried
Golden Kiwifruit	Like	Dislike	Never Tried	White Nectarines	Like	Dislike	Never Tried
Lemons	Like	Dislike	Never Tried	White Peaches	Like	Dislike	Never Tried
Mangoes	Like	Dislike	Never Tried	Brown Pears	Like	Dislike	Never Tried
Nectarines	Like	Dislike	Never Tried				
Oranges	Like	Dislike	Never Tried	**Blue/Purple Fruits:**			
Papayas	Like	Dislike	Never Tried	Blackberries	Like	Dislike	Never Tried
Peaches	Like	Dislike	Never Tried	Blueberries	Like	Dislike	Never Tried
Yellow Pears	Like	Dislike	Never Tried	Black Currants	Like	Dislike	Never Tried
Persimmons	Like	Dislike	Never Tried	Concord Grapes	Like	Dislike	Never Tried
Pineapples	Like	Dislike	Never Tried	Dried Plums	Like	Dislike	Never Tried
Tangerines	Like	Dislike	Never Tried	Elderberries	Like	Dislike	Never Tried
Yellow Watermelon	Like	Dislike	Never Tried	100% Grape Juice	Like	Dislike	Never Tried
				Purple Figs	Like	Dislike	Never Tried
				Purple Grapes	Like	Dislike	Never Tried
				Plums	Like	Dislike	Never Tried
				Raisins	Like	Dislike	Never Tried
Spices							
Black Pepper	Like	Dislike	Never Tried	Parsley	Like	Dislike	Never Tried
Garlic	Like	Dislike	Never Tried	Thyme	Like	Dislike	Never Tried
Ginger	Like	Dislike	Never Tried	Rosemary	Like	Dislike	Never Tried
Crushed Red Pepper	Like	Dislike	Never Tried	Sage	Like	Dislike	Never Tried
Dill	Like	Dislike	Never Tried	Oregano	Like	Dislike	Never Tried
Cayenne Pepper	Like	Dislike	Never Tried	Basil	Like	Dislike	Never Tried
Mint	Like	Dislike	Never Tried	Cumin	Like	Dislike	Never Tried
Paprika	Like	Dislike	Never Tried	Vanilla	Like	Dislike	Never Tried
Turmeric	Like	Dislike	Never Tried	Cocoa	Like	Dislike	Never Tried
Cilantro	Like	Dislike	Never Tried	Mustard	Like	Dislike	Never Tried
						Which One(s)?	
Other Spices		Like	Dislike		Never Tried		

Lean Proteins				If Liked, Which Types?
Fresh fish (Cod, sole, tilapia, trout, tuna, salmon, halibut, flounder, mahi mahi, catfish)	Like	Dislike	Never Tried	
Fresh shellfish (clams, scallops, shrimp, crab, lobster, etc.)	Like	Dislike	Never Tried	
Chicken breast	Like	Dislike	Never Tried	
Turkey breast	Like	Dislike	Never Tried	
Grass-fed beef	Like	Dislike	Never Tried	
Lean cuts of beef: Top sirloin, top/bottom/eye round, round tip	Like	Dislike	Never Tried	
Lean cuts of pork	Like	Dislike	Never Tried	
Wild game such as buffalo, venison, ostrich, etc.	Like	Dislike	Never Tried	
Low-fat milk	Like	Dislike	Never Tried	
Low-fat cheeses: String cheese, ricotta, etc.	Like	Dislike	Never Tried	
Low-fat yogurt	Like	Dislike	Never Tried	
Low-fat cottage cheese	Like	Dislike	Never Tried	
Soy-milk	Like	Dislike	Never Tried	
Eggs	Like	Dislike	Never Tried	
Egg Whites	Like	Dislike	Never Tried	
Cold-Processed Whey Protein	Like	Dislike	Never Tried	
Beans & Lentils (black, black eyed, soy, lima, pinto, split peas, kidney, chickpeas, etc.)	Like	Dislike	Never Tried	
Nuts	Like	Dislike	Never Tried	
Nut Butters	Like	Dislike	Never Tried	

Healthy Fats				If Liked, Which Types?
Olive Oil and Olives	Like	Dislike	Never Tried	
Flax Oil and Flaxseeds	Like	Dislike	Never Tried	
Other Vegetable Oils	Like	Dislike	Never Tried	
Raw Nuts (cashews, almonds, walnuts, pecans, pistachio)	Like	Dislike	Never Tried	
Raw Seeds (pumpkin, sunflower, sesame, chia)	Like	Dislike	Never Tried	
Natural Peanut Butter	Like	Dislike	Never Tried	
Almond Butter	Like	Dislike	Never Tried	
Avocado	Like	Dislike	Never Tried	
Hummus	Like	Dislike	Never Tried	
Fatty Fish (salmon, mackerel, herring, sardines)	Like	Dislike	Never Tried	
Lower Calorie Dressings & Salsa	Like	Dislike	Never Tried	
In Moderation:				
Coconut Oil and Coconuts	Like	Dislike	Never Tried	
Butter	Like	Dislike	Never Tried	
Reduced Fat Cream Cheese	Like	Dislike	Never Tried	
Reduced Fat Sour Cream	Like	Dislike	Never Tried	
Reduced Fat Cheese	Like	Dislike	Never Tried	

Date: ___

How many glasses (8 Fl. Oz) of water did you drink today? ___ [Regular Poland Spring bottle = 2 glasses]

What habit are you tracking? ___

When did you go to bed? ___ Wake-up? ___

Time Start & End (How Fast?)	Place	Food / Beverage (+ condiments, toppings, etc.)	Portion Size	Hunger Rating Key 1 = Starving 10 = Stuffed Hunger Level (Before & After)	Energy Rating Key 1 = Crashing 10 = Feeling Great Energy Level (Before & After)	Stress Rating Key 1 = Totally Relaxed 10 = High Stress Stress Level (Before & After)	Your Habit Specifics: Fruit & Veggie Eaten, Beverage Grade or Indulgence Level

wellness JM

Fruit and Veggie Eating Tracker

Date	Time	Place	Food/Beverage Eaten	Fruit or Veggie Eaten & Portion Size	If No Fruit or Veggie Eaten, How Could You Add One?
1/1/2012	3 PM	At Work	Turkey Sandwich with lettuce, tomato and mustard. Carrots on the side.	One slice of lettuce, two slices tomato. 1/2 cup (handful) of carrots.	Could have a piece of fruit with lunch too.

Beverage Tracking Journal/Assessment

Target Daily Fluid Intake = Half Your Body Weight in Ounces (plus more for exercise)

My Target Daily Fluid Intake = _____ (insert body weight) / 2 = _____ ounces per day

A regular Poland Spring bottle of water equals about 16 ounces of fluid.

Date	Time	Beverage Drank	Added Items (Milk, Sugar, etc.)	Beverage Size (in ounces or approx. size)	Beverage "Grade"
1/1/2012	10:00 AM	Coffee	3 Sugars, Whole Milk	Grande - 16 oz.	B

Beverage Grading System

The beverage grading system has been based on the approximate nutrient density of the different beverages. In general, the best drinks have the least calories and the most naturally-occurring nutrients (i.e. no vitamins artificially added).

• Water or other naturally low-calorie beverages are best.
• There are a number of higher calorie beverages that have some nutrients such as dairy and juice, that can be drank in moderation. For juice, remember you can always have the fruit.
• Then there is a group of drinks that provide a lot of calories and very little nutrients such as soda, sweetened iced tea, fruid drinks, etc.
• Sports drinks can be considered useless calories unless you are refueling yourself during intense physical activity.

The goal of this grading scale is to provide an approximate roadmap as to where your current beverage habits are and how you can possibly improve them (think better grades!). You could probably argue that a certain beverage should be a little higher or lower in the scale and that's fine.

Grade	Beverage
A+	Water
A	Seltzer (not artificially sweetened; see diet beverages)
A	Unsweetened Tea, Green Tea, Iced Tea
A-	Coffee (2 or less sugar packets and a splash of milk)
B+ to C	Smoothies*
B	Soy Milk
B	Skim Milk
B	Low-Fat Milk
B	Coffee (with 3 to 4 sugar packets or lots of milk)
B	Espresso-Based Coffee Drinks without Lots of Sugar (i.e. Cappucino, Latte)
B	Drinks with less than 40 calories per 8 oz. serving (read "servings per container" on the food label)
C	Coffee (with more than 4 packets of sugar and lots of milk)
C	100% Fruit Juice
C	Whole Milk
C-	Sports Drink (unless during intense physical activity, then ok)
C-	Sweetened, Nutrient Enhanced Waters
C-	Blended Coffee Drinks (Mocha/Frappe/Lattes)
C-	Diet Beverages (incl. Diet Soda)
D	Beer
D	Wine
D	Mixed Drink with Low Calorie Mixer
F	Soda
F	Energy Drinks
F	Mixed Drink with High Calorie Mixer
F	Sweetened, Commercial Fruit Drinks
F	Sweetened, Commercial Iced Teas
F	Sweetened, Commercial Lemonades

* The grade of smoothies depend on how processed and how much sugar is added. Whole-food based smoothies are a great post-workout option (i.e. frozen fruit, protein (dairy/soy/vegan), water until desired consistency and maybe some peanut or almond butter).

Indulgence Frequency Assessment

Food	How Much?	How Often?						Alternatives
	Flavor, type, portion size, amount	Monthly	Weekly	A Few Days per Week	Most Days per Week	Daily	Multiple Per Day (How Many?)	Use Preferred Healthy Foods List
Meat								
Hot Dogs								
Hamburgers (non-lean)								
Turkeyburger (non-lean)								
Regular (non-lean) ground beef								
Regular (non-lean) ground turkey								
Bologna								
Salami								
Other High Fat Deli Meats (Salami, Pepperoni, Prosciutto, etc.)								
Sausage								
Bacon								
Ribs								
Juicy Steaks (T-Bone, Strip, etc.)								
Canned Meat								
Starches								
White Bread								
White Pasta								
White Rice								
Flour Tortillas								
White Sandwich Buns/Rolls								
Croutons								
Pretzels								

256

Food	How Much?	How Often?					Alternatives
	Flavor, type, portion size, amount	Monthly	Weekly	A Few Days per Week	Most Days per Week	Daily	Multiple Per Day (How Many?)	Use Preferred Healthy Foods List
Starches, cont'd.								
Chips (Potato, Corn, etc.)								
Loaded Mashed Potatoes								
Macaroni and Cheese								
Pizza								
Sugary Cereals, particularly those with > 10g of Sugar per serving								
* Bread crumbs, croutons, and other dried bread products								
Instant foods (Cake Mixes, Mashed Potatoes, Hamburger Helper)								
Buttery/Processed Popcorn								
Crackers								
Waffles								
Pancakes								
Muffins								
Croissants								
Cake								
Cookies								
Bagels								
Cinnamon Roll								
Doughnuts								
Biscuits								
Regular or low-fat cookies								
Other Starches:								
Other Baked Goods:								

Food	How Much?	How Often?						Alternatives
	Flavor, type, portion size, amount	Monthly	Weekly	A Few Days per Week	Most Days per Week	Daily	Multiple Per Day (How Many?)	Use Preferred Healthy Foods List
Fats								
Half and Half/Cream (in Coffee?)								
Whole-Fat Cream Cheese								
Butter								
Animal Fat/Lard								
Shortening								
Mayonnaise								
Creamy Sauces								
Creamy Dressings								
Creamy Gravies								
Dairy/Eggs								
Whole Eggs (An omelette usually has 3 eggs)								
Whole-Fat Cheese								
Whole Milk								
Ice Cream								
Beverages								
Soda								
Juices								
Fruit Flavored Drinks								
Beer								
Sweetened Iced Tea or Lemonade								
Wine								
Liquor / Mixed Drinks								
Frozen Alcohol Drinks								

Food	How Much? Flavor, type, portion size, amount	How Often? Monthly	Weekly	A Few Days per Week	Most Days per Week	Daily	Multiple Per Day (How Many?)	Alternatives Use Preferred Healthy Foods List
Beverages, cont'd.								
High Calorie Non-Alcohol Drinks (i.e. Frappucinos & Mocha Lattes)								
Tonic Water								
Egg Nog								
Nutrient-Enhanced Waters / Gatorade (unless exercising > 60 mins)								
Fried Foods:								
Fried Chicken								
Fried Fish								
French Fries								
Hashbrowns								
Other Fried Foods								
Dessert/Candy:								
Hard Candies								
Chocolate								
Gummies								
Fruit Snacks								
Fruit canned in syrup								
Candy Bars								
Pudding								
Jello								
Added Sugar / Sugar Packets								
Other Desserts/Candies:								

Food	How Much?	How Often?					Alternatives
	Flavor, type, portion size, amount	Monthly	Weekly	A Few Days per Week	Most Days per Week	Daily	Multiple Per Day (How Many?)	Use Preferred Healthy Foods List
Processed Foods:								
Highly Processed Foods with Lots of Unrecognizeable Ingredients like Lunchables, Pop Tarts, Cheez Whiz								
Ramen/Packaged Noodles								
Non-Lean Packaged Dinners								
Non-Lean Frozen Dinners								
Mixed Dishes with any other Indulgences Listed								
Restaurant Dishes with any other Indulgences Listed								
Restaurant Dishes with More Than 600 calories per plate or 1,000 calories per entire meal								
Take-out or restaurant leftovers								
Other Indulgences Not Listed:								

Indulgence Frequency & Details Tracker

Date	Time	Indulgence Intensity	Food/Drink Eaten	Satisfaction Gained	Reason for Indulgence	How to Prevent If Not Desired
1/1/2012	3 PM	4	3 Cookies	3	Stress, Boredom at Work	Bring My Afternoon Snack

Key:

1. Indulgence Intensity (with examples)	
Level 2 =	Couple cookies, scoop of ice cream, alcoholic drink, can of soda, etc.
Level 5 =	A big dessert, a few drinks,
Level 8 =	Heavy drinking, high-calorie meal or major snack like pint of ice cream
Level 10 =	Lots of drinking + eating, a huge multicourse meal or a binge (sheath of cookies, half pizza)
2. Food / Drink Eaten	
Write down what you ate/drank for your indulgence	

3. Satisfaction Gained
How much did you enjoy the indulgence? Was it planned? How did you feel afterward? 1 = Unhappy, Guilt / 10 = Enjoyed, Appreciated
4. Reason for Indulgence
What caused you to indulge? Were you planning it? Or was it boredom, stress, emotions, etc.?
5. How to Prevent, If Not Desired
If you did not want to indulge, how can you prevent it from happening in the future?

Weekly Physical Activity Tracker

JM wellness

Week of:	Planned Physical Activities	Duration of Each Activity	Intensity 1 = Extremely Easy 10 = Totally Exhausting	Hours Seated (Habit #7)	Daily Steps Taken (Habit #8)	Bedtime	Wake-Up
Monday							
Tuesday							
Wednesday							
Thursday							
Friday							
Saturday							
Sunday							

Easy Eight Strategies Worksheet

Current Results = Current Eating Habits + Current Physical Activity + Current Lifestyle
One small change can go a long way...so based on your current habits:

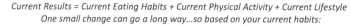

1. **Habit 1: Eat More Often – Eat one more meal/balanced snack per day**

   At home:

   At work:

   On the weekend

   Away from home/Traveling:

   Other:

2. **Habit 2: Eat Smaller Meals – Eat a bit less at meals (80-90%)**

   At home:

   At work:

   On the weekend/away from home:

   Away from home/Traveling:

   Other:

3. **Habit 3: Eat More Fruits and Veggies – Four more per week**

   At home:

   At work:

   On the weekend/away from home:

   Away from home/Traveling:

   Other:

4. **Habit 4: Drink More Low- or No-Calorie Beverages – Or replace high calorie beverages**

   At home:

   At work:

   On the weekend/away from home:

   Away from home/Traveling:

   Other:

5. **Habit 5: Indulge Less Frequently – Have one or two less indulgences each week**

   At home:

   At work:

   On the weekend/away from home:

   Away from home/Traveling:

   Other:

6. **Habit 6: Increase Your Physical Activity – One more day or 30 more minutes each week**

   At home:

   At work:

   On the weekend/away from home:

   Away from home/Traveling:

   Other:

7. **Habit 7: Sit Less – One less hour per day**

   At home:

   At work:

   On the weekend/away from home:

   Away from home/Traveling:

   Other:

8. **Habit 8: Walk More – Take 500 to 1000 more steps each day (5 to 10 city blocks)**

   At home:

   At work:

   On the weekend/away from home:

   Away from home/Traveling:

   Other:

Weekly Evaluation Template

Week of:	My Whys:	My Health, Fitness or Weight Change Desires:		
		My Current Target Easy Eight Habit Change(s):		
	How I Accomplished Today's Easy Eight Habit	How I Will Accomplish Tomorrow's Easy Eight habit	Today's Achievements	Tomorrow's Top Three "To-Do's"	Problem Solving / Improvement Opp's
Monday					
Tuesday					
Wednesday					
Thursday					
Friday					
Saturday					
Sunday					

265

My Energy Tracking Journal

Date	Time	Energy Level	Food Selection/Timing	Way to Boost Energy in Future
1/1/2012	3 PM	3	Small salad at lunch at 12 PM, nothing since	Have a soup with lunch or keep an afternoon snack with me.

Key:
1. Energy Level
1 = Completely Wiped, 10 = Fantastic
2. Food Selection
If Energy is Less than a 4, write down the last time you ate and what it was
3. Way to Boost Energy in Future
Idea how to prevent a low energy level at this time in the future

My Hunger Tracking Journal

Date	Time	Hunger Level	Food Selection/Timing	Way to Decrease Hunger in Future
1/1/2012	3 PM	2	Only small salad at lunch at 12 PM...overate dinner at 8 PM	Make sure to keep my snack with me at 4 PM

Key:
1. Hunger Level
1 = Starving, 10 = Stuffed
2. Food Selection
If Hunger is a 3 or Less, write down the last time you ate and what it was
3. Ways to Reduce Hunger in Future
Ideas how to prevent becoming ravenous at this time in the future

My Stress Tracking Journal

Date	Time	Stress Level	What's causing the stress and how does it make me feel?	How can I handle the stress in a positive way? Or solve it?
1/1/2012	5:00 PM	7	A last-minute deadline at work just as I was getting ready to leave. I felt irritated. Once I finished felt like I deserved something sweet for my hard work.	I knew I hadn't eaten in a while so I was both hungry and irritated. I felt the pang for cookies. But then I stopped & took five deep breaths to clear my mind. I decided to go with a granny smith apple instead and was satisfied.

Key:
1. Stress Level
1 = Relaxed, 10 = Out of control
2. Stress Cause & Feeling
Consider what is stressing you out and if it is making you crave something.
3. Handling or Solving Stress
What actions can you take to deal with or solve the stressful situation.

GREENS RECIPES

GROOVY GREEN SMOOTHIE

http://allrecipes.com/Recipe/Groovy-Green-Smoothie/Detail.aspx

OMELET WITH TURNIP GREENS, GOAT CHEESE & CHILI

http://dutchfood.about.com/od/mainmeals/r/OmeletTurnipTop.htm

GRILLED ENDIVE WITH CHIPOTLE YOGURT DRESSING

http://www.eliseskitchen.com/?p=476

BALSAMIC-GRILLED RADICCHIO WITH SHAVED PECORINO

http://www.epicurious.com/recipes/food/views/Balsamic-Grilled-Radicchio-with-Shaved-Pecorino-232705

ASIAN RADISH GREENS PASTA SAUCE OVER SOBA NOODLES

http://millicanfarms.farmpage.org/2011/04/11/asian-radish-greens-pasta-sauce-over-soba-noodles/

PASTA WITH GREENS AND TOMATO SAUCE

http://www.eatingwell.com/recipes/pasta_with_greens_tomato_sauce.html

GOAT CHEESE AND THREE GREENS LASAGNA

http://www.shape.com/dinner/goat-cheese-and-three-greens-lasagna

LENTIL AND GREEN COLLARD SOUP

http://allrecipes.com/Recipe/Lentil-and-Green-Collard-Soup/Detail.aspx

TUSCAN BEAN SOUP

http://www.foodnetwork.com/recipes/emeril-lagasse/tuscan-bean-soup-recipe/index.html

SHREDDED KALE SALAD

http://theradioblog.marthastewart.com/wp-content/uploads/2010/03/radioblog_recipes_shredded_kale_salad3.pdf

SAUTÉED GREENS WITH PINE NUTS AND RAISINS

http://simplyrecipes.com/recipes/sauteed_greens_with_pine_nuts_and_raisins/

SWEET AND SAVORY SWISS CHARD WRAP

http://www.recipesforkidschallenge.com/submissions/823-sweet-and-savory-swiss-chard-wraps

MEDIATOR RELEASE TEST (MRT) AND LIFESTYLE EATING AND PERFORMANCE (LEAP) THERAPY LINKS

LEAP DISEASE MANAGEMENT WEBSITE: *http://www.nowleap.com/index.html*

LEAP PATIENTS: *http://www.nowleap.com/leap_patients/index.html*

ALLERGY TESTING & LEAP: *http://www.healthydirectionspoway.com/how-can-a-registered-dietician-and-certified-leap-therapist-help-you/allergy-testing-leap*

BOOKS AND PROGRAMS FOR MAKING POSITIVE CHANGES IN ALL SEVEN DIMENSIONS OF WELLNESS

JACK CANFIELD – THE SUCCESS PRINCIPLES: *http://www.thesuccessprinciples.com*

AMANDA CARLSON-PHILLIPS – CORE PERFORMANCE: *http://www.coreperformance.com*

KEN BLANCHARD & SPENCER JOHNSON – ONE MINUTE MANAGER: *http://www.kenblanchard.com*

DAVID BACH – THE AUTOMATIC MILLIONAIRE: *http://www.finishrich.com*

SHAWN ACHOR – THE HAPPINESS ADVANTAGE: *http://www.shawnachor.com*

CHARLES DUHIGG – THE POWER OF HABIT: *http://www.charlesduhigg.com/the-power-of-habit*

CHIP AND DAN HEATH – SWITCH: *http://www.heathbrothers.com/switch*

JOHN BERARDI – PRECISION NUTRITION: *http://www.precisionnutrition.com*

PROFESSIONAL COACHING SERVICES AND LINKS

COACH U: *http://www.coachinc.com/*

INTERNATIONAL COACH FEDERATION: *http://www.coachfederation.org*

ADAM GILBERT – MY BODY TUTOR: *http://www.MyBodyTutor.com*

WELLCOACHES: *http://www.wellcoachesschool.com/*

REFERENCES

CHAPTER 2

Curioni, C. C. and Lourenco, P. M. (2005). Long-term weight loss after diet and exercise: a systematic review. International Journal of Obesity 29: 1168-1174. Accessed on 7/16/12 at: http://www.nature.com/ijo/journal/v29/n10/abs/0803015a.html

Wing, R.R. and Phelan, S. (2005). Long-term weight loss maintenance. American Journal of Clinical Nutrition 82(1): 222S-225S. Accessed on 7/16/12 at: http://www.ajcn.org/content/82/1/222S.short

Valuation of U.S. weight loss market from Marketdata Enterprises. May 9, 2011 at: http://www.prweb.com/releases/2011/5/prweb8393658.htm

LeBlanc E. S. et al. (2011). Effectiveness of primary care – Relevant treatments for obesity in adults: A systematic evidence review for the U.S. preventive services task force. Annals of Internal Medicine 155: 434-447. Accessed on 7/16/12 at: http://www.ncbi.nlm.nih.gov/pubmed/21969342

Tate, D. F., Jacknovy, E. H. and Wing, R. R. (2006). A randomized trial comparing human e-mail counseling, computer-automated tailored counseling and no counseling in an internet weight loss program. Archives of Internal Medicine 166(15): 1620-1625. Accessed on 7/16/12 at: http://archinte.jamanetwork.com/article.aspx?articleid=410781

CHAPTER 3

Inspiration for some aspects of Anspaugh's Seven Dimensions of Wellness descriptions from the Franklin Pierce Wellness Department: http://eraven.franklinpierce.edu/s/dept/hr/Wellness/Wellness_Publications/Seven Dimensions of Wellness.pdf

Find the Seven Dimensions of Wellness from the source: Anspaugh, D. J, Hamrick, M. H., and Rosato, F. D. (2010). Wellness: Concepts and Applications. 8th ed.

Mc-Graw Hill. http://www.amazon.com/Wellness-Concepts-Applications-David-Anspaugh/dp/0078022509

Foster, L. T. (2007). Section 2: Defining wellness and Its determinants. British Columbia Atlas of Wellness. University of Victoria. Accessed on 7/16/12 at: www.geog.uvic.ca/wellness/wellness/2_DefiningWellness.pdf

CHAPTER 4

Oxford Dictionary. (2012). s.v. "Diet." Accessed on 7/16/12 at: http://oxforddictionaries.com/definition/english/diet

Sacks, F. M. et al. (2009). Comparison of weight-loss diets with different compositions of fat, protein and carbohydrates. New England Journal of Medicine. 360: 859-873. Accessed on 7/16/12 at: http://www.nejm.org/doi/full/10.1056/nejmoa0804748

Rossner, S. and Flaten, H. (1997). VLCD versus LCD in long-term treatment of obesity. International Journal of Obesity 21: 22-26. Accessed on 7/16/12 at: http://knowledgetranslation.ca/sysrev/articles/project21/Rossner%20S,%20Int%20J%20Obes%20Relat%20Metab%20Disord.%201997%3B21(1),22-6-20090717112654.pdf

MedicineNet.com. (2003). Weight cycling...Facts about "yo-yo" dieting. Accessed on 7/16/12 at: http://www.medicinenet.com/script/main/art.asp?articlekey=21745

Baye, D. (2010). Q&A: How many calories does a pound of muscle burn? Accessed on 7/16/12 at: http://baye.com/qa-calories-burned-by-muscle/

CHAPTER 7

Schusdziarra, V. et al. (2011). Impact of breakfast on daily energy intake – an analysis of absolute versus relative breakfast calories. Nutrition Journal 10(5). Accessed on 7/16/12 at: http://www.nutritionj.com/content/10/1/5/abstract

Goldstone, A. P. et al. (2009). Fasting biases brain reward systems towards high-calorie foods. European Journal of Neuroscience 30(8): 1625-1635. Accessed on 7/16/12 at: http://onlinelibrary.wiley.com/doi/10.1111/j.1460-9568.2009.06949.x/abstract

Jakubowicz, D. et al. (2012). Meal timing and composition influence ghrelin levels, appetite scores and weight loss maintenance in overweight and obese individuals. Steroids 77(4): 323-331. Accessed on 7/16/12 at: http://www.sciencedirect.com/science/article/pii/S0039128X11003515

National Weight Control Registry. Research findings accessed on 7/16/12 at: http://www.nwcr.ws/Research/default.htm

Wansink, B., van Ittersum, K. and Painter, J. E. (2006). Ice cream illusions: Bowls, spoons, and self-served portion sizes. American Journal of Preventive Medicine 31(3): 240-243. Accessed on 7/16/12 at: http://www.sciencedirect.com/science/article/pii/S0749379706001796

Bite-size pieces research by Devina Wadhera, to be presented at 2012 Annual Meeting of the Society for the Study of Ingestive Behavior (SSIB). Accessed on 7/23/12 at: http://www.foodnavigator.com/Science-Nutrition/Bite-size-foods-are-more-rewarding-suggests-study

Spinach protein value from Nutritiondata.self.com: http://www.calorieking.com/foods/calories-in-fresh-or-dried-vegetables-spinach-raw-edible-portion_f-ZmlkPTcxMDI4.html

Kale nutrient values from Nutritiondata.self.com: http://nutritiondata.self.com/facts/vegetables-and-vegetable-products/2461/2

Donaldson, M. S. (2004). Nutrition and cancer: A review of the evidence for an anti-cancer diet.

Nutrition Journal, 3(19), accessed on 12/10/11 at: http://www.nutritionj.com/content/3/1/19

Kontogianni, M. et al. (2009). Nutrition recommendations and interventions for subjects with cardiovascular disease. Nutrition and Metabolism, Part 4: 221-244. Accessed on 7/16/12 at: http://www.springerlink.com/content/h66mv45m24g661m5/

Jequier, E. and Constant, F. (2010). Water as an essential nutrient: the physiological basis of hydration. European Journal of Clinical Nutrition. 64: 115-123.

American College of Sports Medicine, American Dietetic Association and Dietitians of Canada. (2009). Nutrition and athletic performance. Journal of American Dietetic Association. 109(3): 509-527. Accessed on 7/16/12 at: http://www.ncbi.nlm.nih.gov/sites/entrez/19278045?dopt=Abstract&holding=f1000,f1000m,isrctn.

Lamina, S. and Musa, D. (2009). Ergogenic effect of varied doses of coffee-caffeine on maximal aerobic power of young African subjects. African Health Sciences. 9(4): 270-274. Accessed on 7/16/12 at: http://www.ncbi.nlm.nih.gov/pmc/articles/PMC3074398/

World Anti-Doping Agency. (2012). The world anti-doping code prohibited list: International standard.

Butt, M. S. and Sultan, M. T. (2011). Coffee and its consumption: Benefits and risks. Critical Reviews in Food Science and Nutrition. 51: 363-373.

Snel, J. and Lorist, M. M. (2011). Effects of caffeine on sleep and cognition. Progress in Brain Research. 190: 105-117.

Yang, Q. (2010). Gain weight by "going diet?" Artificial sweeteners and the neurobiology of sugar cravings. Yale Journal of Biology and Medicine. 83(2): 101-108. Accessed on 7/16/12 at: http://www.ncbi.nlm.nih.gov/pmc/articles/PMC2892765/

Applebee's "Oriental grilled chicken" salad nutrition info accessed via: http://applebees.com/~/media/docs/Applebees_Nutritional_Info.ashx on 7/16/2012.

Pelchat, M. L. et al. (2004). Images of desire: food-craving activation during fMRI. NeuroImage. 23(4): 1486-1493. Accessed on 7/16/12 at: http://www.sciencedirect.com/science/article/pii/S1053811904004847

Holpuch, A. & Fitbie (2012). 7 distractions that help cut cravings. Accessed on 7/16/12 at: http://fitbie.msn.com/slideshow/7-distractions-help-cut-cravings/ (I contributed)

Farley, A. C. et al. (2012). "Interventions for preventing weight gain after smoking cessation." Cochrane Tobacco Addiction Group. Accessed on 7/16/12 at: http://onlinelibrary.wiley.com/doi/10.1002/14651858.CD006219.pub3/abstract

Hoebel, B. G. et al. (2009). Natural addiction: A behavioral and circuit model based on sugar addiction in rats. Journal of Addiction Medicine. 3(1): 33-41. Accessed on 7/16/12 at: http://journals.lww.com/journaladdictionmedicine/Abstract/2009/03000/Natural_Addiction__A_Behavioral_and_Circuit_Model.5.aspx

Fitness Education Network. (2012). Section 2: Benefits of regular physical activity. American College of Sports Medicine certified personal trainer workshop study guide. www.FitnessEdNet.com

Saunders, T. (2010). Ten simple ways to increase your physical activity. Accessed on 7/16/12 at: http://scienceblogs.com/obesitypanacea/2010/03/ten_simple_ways_to_increase_yo.php

Tabata, I. et al. (1996). Effects of moderate-intensity endurance and high-intensity intermittent training on anaerobic capacity and VO2 max. Medicine and Science in Sports and Exercise. 28(10): 1327-1330. Accessed on 7/16/12 at: http://www.ncbi.nlm.nih.gov/pubmed/8897392

Ploughman, M. (2008). Exercise is brain food: The effects of physical activity on cognitive function. Developmental Neurorehabilitation. 11(3): 236-240. Accessed on 7/16/12 at: http://informahealthcare.com/doi/abs/10.1080/17518420801997007

Lautenschlager, N. T. et al. (2008). Effect of physical activity on cognitive function in older adults at risk for Alzheimer's disease: A randomized trial. Journal of the American Medical Association. 300(9): 1027-1037. Accessed on 7/16/12 at: http://jama.jamanetwork.com/article.aspx?articleid=182502

Lustig, C. et al. (2009). Aging, training, and the brain: A review and future directions. Neuropsychology Review. 19(4): 504-522. Accessed on 7/16/12 at: http://www.ncbi.nlm.nih.gov/pmc/articles/PMC3005345/

Sitting ergonomics pictures provided by Occupational Safety and Health Administration. Accessed on 7/16/12 at: http://www.osha.gov/SLTC/etools/computerwork-stations/positions.html

Parker-Pope T. "Workplace cited as a new source of rise in obesity." Available at: http://www.nytimes.com/2011/05/26/health/nutrition/26fat.html?pagewanted=all. Accessed July, 17, 2012.

Sitting, standing and walking calorie values based on MET values for a 150 pound individual. Walking is at 2.5 miles per hour. Values obtained from www.CaloriesPerHour.com

American College of Sports Medicine (2011). Quantity and quality of exercise for developing and maintaining cardiorespiratory, musculoskeletal and neuromotor fitness in apparently healthy adults: Guidance for prescribing exercise. Medicine and Science in Sports and Exercise. 43(7): 1334-1359. Accessed on 1/7/12 at: http://journals.lww.com/acsm-msse/Fulltext/2011/07000/Quantity_and_Quality_of_Exercise_for_Developing.26.aspx

CHAPTER 8

Lally, P. et al. (2010). How are habits formed: Modeling habit formation in the real world. European Journal of Social Psychology. 40(6): 998-1009. Accessed on 7/16/12 at: http://onlinelibrary.wiley.com/doi/10.1002/ejsp.674/abstract;jsessionid=24260A73A5AF8195FD24216A31CBE9CE.d02t02

Dallongeville, J. et al. (1998). Cigarette smoking is associated with unhealthy patterns of nutrient intake: a meta-analysis. Journal of Nutrition. 128(9): 1450-1457. Accessed 6/18/11 at: http://jn.nutrition.org/content/128/9/1450.full

Chiolero, A. et al. (2008). Consequences of smoking for body weight, body fat distribution, and insulin resistance. American Journal of Clinical Nutrition. 87(4): 801-809. Accessed on 6/18/11 at: http://www.ajcn.org/content/87/4/801.full

Campaign for Tobacco-Free Kids. (2002). Smoking, physical activity, and poor physical performance. Accessed on 7/16/12 at: www.tobaccofreekids.org/research/factsheets/pdf/0177.pdf

National Institutes of Health. (2007). Stressed out? Stress affects both body and mind. NIH News in Health. January 2007 ed. Accessed on 7/16/12 at: http://newsinhealth.nih.gov/2007/January/docs/01features_01.htm

Chandola, T., Brunner, E. and Marmot, M. (2006). Chronic stress at work and the metabolic syndrome: prospective study. British Medical Journal: 332, 551. Accessed on 7/16/12 at: http://www.bmj.com/content/332/7540/521.full

Torres, S. J. and Nowson, C. A. (2007). Relationship between stress, eating behavior, and obesity. Nutrition: 23(11-12), 887-894. Accessed on 7/16/12 at: http://www.sciencedirect.com/science/article/pii/S0899900707002493

Pike, J. L. et al. (1997). Chronic life stress alters sympathetic, neuroendocrine, and immune responsivity to an acute psychological stressor in humans. Psychosomatic Medicine. 59(4): 447-457. Accessed on 7/16/12 at: http://www.psychosomaticmedicine.org/content/59/4/447.short

Newcomer, J. W. et al. (1999). Decreased memory performance in healthy humans induced by stress-level cortisol treatment. Archives of General Psychiatry. 56(6): 527-533. Accessed on 7/16/12 at: http://ukpmc.ac.uk/abstract/MED/10359467

Lupien, S. J. et al. (2009). Effects of stress throughout the lifespan on the brain, behavior and cognition. Nature Reviews: Neuroscience. 10: 434-445. Accessed on 7/16/12 at: http://www.nature.com/nrn/journal/v10/n6/abs/nrn2639.html

Knutson, K. L. et al. (2007). The metabolic consequences of sleep deprivation. Sleep Medicine Reviews. 11(3): 163-178. Accessed on 7/16/12 at: http://www.sciencedirect.com/science/article/pii/S1087079207000202

Babyak, M. et al. (2000). Exercise treatment for major depression: Maintenance of therapeutic benefit at 10 months. Psychosomatic Medicine. 62(5), 633-638. Accessed on 7/16/12 at: http://www.psychosomaticmedicine.org/content/62/5/633.short

Dunn, A. L. et al. (2005). Exercise treatment for depression: Efficacy and dose response. American Journal of Preventive Medicine. 28(1): 1-8. Accessed on 7/16/12 at: http://www.sciencedirect.com/science/article/pii/S0749379704002417

EPILOGUE

Dr. Bruce Lipton and Subconscious Power: http://www.brucelipton.com/

Michael Gelb and Subconscious Power: How to Think Like Leonardo da Vinci: Seven Steps to Genius Every Day, Published in 2000 by Dell Publishing

INDEX